Geriatric Psychiatry

Review of Psychiatry Series
John M. Oldham, M.D., M.S.
Michelle B. Riba, M.D., M.S.
Series Editors

Geriatric Psychiatry

EDITED BY

Alan M. Mellow, M.D., Ph.D.

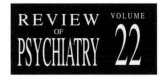

No. 4

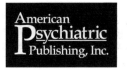

Washington, DC
London, England

Chapter 5
Geriatric Psychiatry at the Crossroads of
Public Policy and Clinical Practice   145

Christopher C. Colenda, M.D, M.P.H.
Stephen J. Bartels, M.D., M.S.
Joel E. Streim, M.D.
Christine deVries

health-promoting habits and behaviors. Because understanding motivated behavior is a mainstay of what psychiatry is all about and we still have not unraveled all of the reasons why humans do things that are bad for them, business will be brisk.

Continuing our tradition of presenting a selection of topics in each year's Review of Psychiatry Series that includes new research findings and new developments in clinical care, we look forward to Volume 23 in the Review of Psychiatry Series, which will feature brain stimulation in psychiatric treatment (edited by Sarah H. Lisanby, M.D.), developmental psychobiology (edited by B. J. Casey, Ph.D.), medical laboratory and neuropsychiatric testing (edited by Stuart C. Yudofsky, M.D., and H. Florence Kim, M.D.), and cognitive-behavioral therapy (edited by Jesse H. Wright III, M.D., Ph.D.).

Preface

Alan M. Mellow, M.D., Ph.D.

In the 1980s and 1990s, geriatricians—whether psychiatrists, psychologists, neurologists, internists or others—were often characterized as "crusaders," fighting for the proper treatment of older patients, who were often neglected. These clincians continually pointed out that the elderly were subject to ageist biases, had many barriers to diagnosis and treatment, and importantly, did not have the benefit of a coherent knowledge base to inform clinical practice, because the elderly had been excluded from much of the mainstream clinical research that had moved medicine forward so dramatically in the past several decades. Although many of the barriers to good care for the elderly remain, and most of us in geriatrics still wear our "crusader" mantles, considerable progress has been made. With the aging of the population, the demographic imperative is now well-accepted by all. In geriatric psychiatry, a deeper understanding of the neurobiology of aging, as well as a growing knowledge base from fields as wide ranging as molecular biology, genetics, neuroimaging, pharmacology, and health services research has yielded what we attempt to overview in this volume of the *Review of Psychiatry* series.

In Chapter 1, my colleagues Drs. Kales and Maixner and I review the most common syndromes in geriatric psychiatry, those of late-life depression and anxiety. We also consider the increasing body of knowledge on what is now recognized as a significant clinical problem, that of depression complicating dementia. In Chapter 2, Dr. Weiner presents an overview of dementia itself, including what has been learned recently about the non-Alzheimer's dementias such as dementia with Lewy bodies and frontotemporal dementias. He also reviews the latest data on established and experimental treatments for Alzheimer's disease. Drs. Grossberg and Desai, in their chapter on late-life psychoses (Chapter 3),

(Blazer et al. 1986), supported by other evidence that the incidence of depression is increasing (Klerman and Weissman 1989). This latter finding has recently been challenged by the Stirling County study, which showed a stable prevalence of depression over a 40-year period (Murphy et al. 2000).

The issues of strictly diagnosed major depression in community studies notwithstanding, subsyndromal depressive symptoms may be as high as 15%–25% (Koenig and Blazer 1992) in the community. In primary care patients, the prevalence of major depression is 10%–15% (Katon and Schulberg 1992; Schulberg et al. 1999). This rate rises to 15%–20% in long-term care settings, and for subsyndromal depressive symptoms it rises to as high as 40% (Parmelee et al. 1989; Rovner et al. 1986). Because functional disability is associated with both major depression and depressive symptoms (Lyness et al. 1999, 2002; Rovner and Ganguli 1998; Wells et al. 1989), these prevalence rates represent what many would argue is a major public health problem as the population ages.

Recognition and Diagnosis of Depression in Older Patients

For the most part, DSM-IV-TR (American Psychiatric Association 2000) criteria are applicable to major depression in late life, but elderly patients can present with atypical syndromes, making diagnosis more problematic. Older patients may present with anhedonia and somatic complaints and without depressed mood (Gallo and Rabins 1999). In addition, the presence of comorbid medical illness may complicate the symptom picture (Cohen-Cole and Stoudemire 1987; Kathol et al. 1990). The presence of coexisting cognitive impairment and depression is discussed in detail later. These factors are all of particular importance because most older patients with depression are not seen by mental health professionals, but rather are seen exclusively by primary care providers (Cole and Yaffe 1996; Ganguli et al. 1995), and depression is underdiagnosed and undertreated by these providers (Perez-Stable et al. 1990; Wells et al. 1989). Recent efforts have focused on training and support programs to aid primary care providers in better diagnosing and treating geriatric depression (G. Livingston et al. 2000; Philip 1998).

Treatment

Antidepressants

In light of the concerns about adequate recognition of depression in older patients, particularly in the primary care setting, it is encouraging to note that most research supports treatment responses to antidepressant therapy in older patients comparable with that seen in younger cohorts (Bressler and Katz 1993; Gerson et al. 1988). In studies comparing older tricyclic antidepressants (TCAs) to the newer selective serotonin reuptake inhibitors (SSRIs; Schneider 1996), SSRIs have shown, for the most part, equal efficacies and superior side effect profiles (Mulsant et al. 2001; Schneider 1996), making them current first-line pharmacotherapy for geriatric depression. Efficacy has been demonstrated in this patient group for bupropion (Branconnier et al. 1983), venlafaxine (Staab and Evans 2000), and mirtazapine (Schatzberg et al. 2002).

Psychotherapy

Psychotherapeutic approaches—primarily cognitive-behavioral therapy (CBT) and interpersonal therapies—have been demonstrated to be efficacious in geriatric depression both alone and in combination with antidepressant treatment (Karel and Hinrichsen 2000; Klausner and Alexopoulos 1999; Niederehe 1996). In addition to acute treatment, psychotherapy has a role in the long-term maintenance treatment of depression in the elderly (Reynolds et al. 1995).

Depression in Dementia

The interface of depression and dementia is a challenging but critical area in the assessment and treatment of both disorders. The traditional focus of this interface has been an emphasis on avoiding the misdiagnosis of dementia in elderly patients who

Dexamethasone Suppression Test (DST) in 10 of 20 patients with dementia; nonsuppressors had significantly higher depression scores on the Depressive Signs Scale (DSS) than did supressors. Following antidepressant treatment, three of eight nonsuppressors reverted to normal suppression, but this was not associated with clinical improvement.

Assessment

Because they have symptoms in common, depression sometimes can be misdiagnosed as dementia (pseudodementia) and vice versa (pseudodepression). These overlap symptoms are generally more chronic and slowly developing in dementia and more subacute in depression. Depression and apathy or lack of motivation associated with dementia may also be difficult to distinguish from depression in some cases. It is estimated that apathy is experienced by 40%–50% of patients with early or intermediate AD (Rubin et al. 1987), 10% of patients with left-hemisphere stroke, and 25% of patients with right-hemisphere stroke (Marin et al. 1994; Starkstein et al. 1993). Apathy and depression often coexist; one recent study found that 37% of AD patients studied had apathy—24% with depression and 13% with no depression (Starkstein et al. 2001).

The possibility of a superimposed depression in dementia should be considered when chronic symptoms associated with dementia progression such as weight loss, sleep changes due to loss of diurnal rhythms, or amotivation become more severe over the course of a few weeks (Thorpe and Groulx 2001). In terms of specific symptoms seen in major depression in dementia, depressed patients with dementia have been found to have symptom profiles similar to those of patients without dementia (Chemerinski et al. 2001; Cummings 1988), especially in mild dementia (Draper 1999).

Pseudodementia

Historically, much emphasis has been given to the distinction of depression from dementia in late-life. The term *pseudodementia* has long been used to denote the cognitive impairment that occurs with depression and reverses with adequate treatment of mood symptoms. However, more recent studies have revealed that many cases of pseudodementia either have cognitive deficits that do not remit despite clinical recovery (Abas et al. 1990) or are found to have irreversible cognitive impairment on follow-up (Alexopoulos et al. 1993). In one study, up to 50% of geriatric patients with "reversible dementia" were found to have irreversible dementia at 5-year follow-up (Alexopoulos et al. 1993). Butters et al. (2000) found that elderly nondemented subjects with depression and mild cognitive impairment improved cognitively with remission of mood symptoms but remained mildly cognitively impaired. These authors noted that this subgroup of late-life depression patients is likely at high risk of developing progressive dementia.

These findings have led some to suggest that pseudodementia may in fact be "predementia" (Reifler 2000), although a small study of subjects who died during a major depressive episode did not confirm that cognitive impairment during a depressive episode was related to AD or vascular dementia–type neuropathological change on autopsy (O'Brien et al. 2001). A recent small single photon emission computed tomography (SPECT) study of depressive pseudodementia subjects compared with healthy control subjects, depressed subjects, and AD subjects found decreased cerebral blood flow in the psuedodementia group in the temporoparietal region, similar to that of the AD group and different from that of the depression group (Cho et al. 2002). Taking into account the studies to date suggests that, in a subset of elderly patients (perhaps up to half), depression heralds a dementia syndrome. These lines of evidence have led investigators to study the question of whether depression is a prodromal symptom of dementia or whether it might be an actual risk factor for dementia.

Provisional Diagnostic Criteria

Recently, a group of investigators with extensive research and clinical experience related to late-life depression and AD proposed provisional diagnostic criteria for depression in AD for the purpose of 1) facilitating hypothesis-driven research in this area

Table 1–1. Placebo-controlled outcomes trials for depression dementia

Author	Antidepressant	Method	Outcomes	Comments
Reifler et al. (1989)	Imipramine (TCA)	8 week trial HRSD, MMSE, DRS, OARS ratings Therapeutic imipramine levels	Significant but comparable improvement in imipramine and placebo groups	Worsened cognition (DRS scores) in imipramine group possible due to anticholinergic effect of imipramine
Petracca et al. (1996)	Clomipramine (TCA)	HRSD, MMSE	Significant improvement in clomipramine and placebo groups Significantly greater mood improvement with clomipramine	MMSE score improved more during clomipramine crossover to placebo (?more adverse cognitive effects of clomipramine)
Roth et al. (1996)	Moclobemide (reversible MAOI)	6 week trial HRSD, MMSE, SCAG, GDS	Significant improvement in moclobemide and placebo groups Significantly greater mood improvement with moclobemide	No cognitive effects of moclobemide noted

Table 1–1. Placebo-controlled outcomes trials for depression dementia (*continued*)

Author	Antidepressant	Method	Outcomes	Comments
Lyketsos et al. (2000b)	Sertraline (SSRI)	12 week trial CSDD, HRSD, MMSE	Significantly more clinical improvement in sertraline group Significantly more partial responders in sertraline group	No cognitive effects of sertraline noted

Note. CSDD = Cornell Scale for Depression in Dementia; DRS = Dementia Rating Scale; GDS = Geriatric Depression Scale; HRSD = Hamilton Rating Scale for Depression; MAOI = monoamine oxidase inhibitor; MMSE = Mini-Mental State Examination; OARS = Older Americans' Resources and Services Assessment Scale; SCAG = Sandoz Clinical Assessment–Geriatric; SSRI = selective serotonin re-uptake inhibitor; TCA = tricyclic antidepressant.

Interpersonal and Behavioral Approaches

As noted in Table 1–1, significant placebo response has been found in three of the four placebo-controlled trials. Katz (1998) noted that the pronounced improvement of depressive symptoms in placebo groups in those trials suggests that interpersonal or behavioral approaches might be effective in the treatment of depression in dementia. Teri et al. (1997) studied two types of behavioral interventions, the use of pleasant events for patients living in the community and teaching problem solving for patients' caregivers compared with a control wait-list condition in depressed patients with AD. Both approaches were associated with significant improvement in depressive symptoms both in patients and caregivers, and the improvement was maintained for 6 months. These results suggest that treatment of the caregiver may be an important factor in the treatment of the patient or that providing some type of supportive intervention improves the patient–caregiver dyad.

Anxiety in Late Life

Anxiety disorders are the most common diagnosable conditions in older adults (Blazer et al. 1991). However, anxiety in the elderly is one of the least studied areas of geriatric psychiatry. Little research has been conducted on how anxiety disorders' presentation and comorbidity differ in older adults as compared with younger persons or on the treatment of anxiety in the older adult. Just as for depression in older adults, anxiety increases health service utilization and costs (Blazer et al. 1991). Finally, late-life anxiety symptoms must always evoke an investigation for underlying comorbid medical and psychiatric illness, including substance abuse.

In this section, we provide an overview of the community-based epidemiological studies of these disorders, the specific anxiety disorders with a geriatric focus, and the treatment of anxiety in the elderly.

Epidemiology

Studies show the prevalence of anxiety disorders is lower for the elderly than for other age groups. However, these continue to be the most prevalent group of psychiatric disorders in the geriatric population. Blazer et al. (1991) reported data on the National Institute of Mental Health's Epidemiologic Catchment Area (ECA) Project at Duke University, in which the 3,000–4,000 elderly subjects were surveyed and oversampled. In community samples 65 years of age and older, there was a 6-month prevalence of all anxiety disorders of 19.7% and a lifetime prevalence of 34.05%. This is lower than the younger age group of 45–64, but still notable.

The Berlin Aging Study (BASE; Schaub and Linden 2000) researched anxiety symptoms in 258 community-dwelling and institutionalized younger-old (70–84 years), and 258 very old (85–103 years) persons. Of those studies, 4.3% of the younger group and 2.3% of the older group had clinically significant anxiety. About half met criteria for a specific anxiety disorder, and half were classified as having an anxiety disorder not otherwise specified. Anxiety was more common in females. The most common comorbidities were mood disorders. The BASE authors argued that anxiety disorders in the old are less common than other psychiatric disorders in this age group.

The Guy's/Age Concern Survey of urban-living persons over age 64 found that 3.7% of the subjects studied had generalized anxiety disorder (GAD) and 10.0% had phobic disorders (Lindesay et al. 1989). The Longitudinal Aging Study of Amsterdam (LASA) studied 3,107 patients aged 55–85 and found an overall 6-month prevalence of anxiety disorders of 10.2% (Beekman et al. 1998). The prevalence of GAD was 7.3%, phobic disorders 3.1%, panic disorder 1%, and obsessive-compulsive disorder (OCD) 0.6%. Neither the ECA study, Guys/Age, LASA, nor BASE studies reported on posttraumatic stress disorder (PTSD); however, for many survivors of trauma, symptoms may last decades. Flint (1994) and Krasucki et al. (1998) offered comprehensive reviews of the epidemiology of anxiety disorders in the elderly.

Panic Disorder

Panic disorder is much less common in older persons than younger persons. The 6-month prevalence of panic disorder according to the Duke ECA study is 0.04% in persons 65 years and older, with a lifetime prevalence of 0.29%, much less than that of

case reports have suggested PTSD symptoms may herald onset of a dementia (Johnston 2000; Mittal et al. 2001). Dementia patients with PTSD, in one study, did not differ in behavioral disturbances from control dementia patients but were prescribed more antidepressants. A prisoner-of-war (POW) group studied had more paranoia and less verbal agitation than non-POW patients with PTSD (Verma et al. 2001).

Symptoms of PTSD are similar among older and younger patients. In some studies, younger veterans had higher scores on all PTSD symptoms than older veterans. The older veterans' predominant symptoms were decreased interest in activities and distress from exposure to trauma-related events (Hyer et al. 1995). Older adults may have more somatic symptoms with PTSD (Lipton and Schaffer 1988). Older persons potentially can experience all PTSD symptoms, and more research is needed to clarify a symptom profile unique to older adults, if one indeed exists. There may be differences in profiles depending on the type of trauma. Other factors influencing the development of PTSD may include prior trauma and societal factors (Hautamaki and Coleman 2001).

The Duke ECA community sample did not measure prevalence of PTSD in older adult populations. Prevalence rates from studies of combat veterans of WWII and Korea range from 3% to 56% (Averill and Beck 2000). Higher rates are reported for prisoners of war and Holocaust survivors. High rates of PTSD were found after the air disaster in Lockerbie, Scotland, with 84% of older adults (versus 100% of younger adults) having symptoms at 1 year and 16% at 3 years (Livingston et al. 1994). A community sample of persons experiencing flooding showed a lifetime PTSD prevalence of 1.1% (none of these were female) (Shore et al. 1989). Approximately 2 years after the Buffalo Creek Dam collapse, the rate of PTSD was 28% among those ages 62–73, similar to the rates for younger adults.

Comorbidities include alcohol abuse, depression, and other anxiety disorders. It is hypothesized that the increased physical comorbidities may be due to long-term overactivity of the hypothalamic-pituitary-adrenal stress axis. When controlled for age, smoking, alcohol use, and body weight, WWII and Korean combat veterans with PTSD had increased arterial, lower gastrointestinal, dermatologic, and musculoskeletal conditions (Schnurr and Spiro 1999).

Generalized Anxiety Disorder

GAD is one of the most common anxiety disorders in older adults. The LASA study reported a 6-month prevalence of 7.3% (Beekman et al. 1998). ECA data for community-dwelling older adults noted a 1.9% 1-month prevalence and a 4.6% lifetime prevalence for GAD, but only 38% of these patients used outpatient behavioral health services in the year prior to interview (Blazer et al. 1991). Depressive symptoms are concurrent 90% of time, especially in older adults (Lindesay et al. 1989). Many symptoms overlap with other medical conditions—pulmonary, neurological, cardiovascular, and endocrine disorders—making diagnosis difficult. Of persons with GAD in a long-term care facility, 60% also had major depressive disorder (Parmelee et al. 1993).

GAD is often a recurrent illness with exacerbations and remissions. Quality of life was subjectively rated by older adults with GAD, who reported a lower quality of life; depression and severe anxiety lowered the reported quality of life, and optimism was associated with reports of a better life satisfaction (Bourland et al. 2000).

Phobias

Phobias are the most common anxiety disorders in all populations in a majority of studies. In the Duke ECA community sample, the 6-month prevalence of simple phobia, social phobia, and agoraphobia was 9.63%, 1.37%, and 5.22%, respectively.

Agoraphobia without panic disorder may be the most common late-onset phobia (Lindesay 1991). Lindesay (1991) compared 60 patients with phobic disorders in an urban geriatric community sample with 60 matched control subjects. Specific fears had an early onset, and social impairment was minimal. Over half the time, agoraphobic fears had an onset after age 65 and were attributed to a traumatic event or physical illness. Older adults with phobias had more visits to primary care physi-

with anxiety who were referred by their general practitioners had significant reductions in anxiety symptoms with CBT. Limitations of these studies include loosely defined anxiety states.

Summary

Considerable progress has been made in the past several years in understanding the characteristics, epidemiology, and treatment response of the most common psychiatric disorders—namely, depression and anxiety—in elderly patients. An explosion of knowledge about comorbid depression and dementia has provided new opportunities to care for the growing population of elderly patients with these disorders. Many challenges remain, particularly in improving the recognition and treatment of late-life depression and in furthering our knowledge base of geriatric anxiety disorders.

References

Aarts P, Op den Velde W, Falger P, et al: Late onset of posttraumatic stress disorder in aging resistance veterans in the Netherlands, in Aging and Posttraumatic Stress Disorder. Edited by Riskin P, Talbott J. Washington, DC, American Psychiatric Press, 1996, pp 53–78

Abas MA, Sahakian BJ, Levy R: Neuropsychological deficits and CT scan changes in elderly depressives. Psychol Med 20:507–520, 1990

Alexopoulos GS: The treatment of depressed demented patients. J Clin Psychiatry 57(suppl 14):14–20, 1996

Alexopoulos GS, Abrams RC, Young RC, et al: Cornell Scale for Depression in Dementia. Biol Psychiatry 23:271–284, 1988a

Alexopoulos GS, Abrams RC, Young RC, et al: Use of the Cornell scale in nondemented patients. J Am Geriatr Soc 36:230–236, 1988b

Alexopoulos GS, Meyers BS, Young RC, et al: The course of geriatric depression with "reversible dementia": a controlled study. Am J Psychiatry 150:1693–1699, 1993

Allen H, Jolley D, Comish J, et al: Depression in dementia: a study of mood in a community sample and referrals to a community service. Int J Geriatr Psychiatry 12:513–518, 1997

American Psychiatric Association: Diagnostic and Statistical Manual of Mental Disorders, 4th Edition, Text Revision. Washington, DC, American Psychiatric Association, 2000

Averill PM, Beck JG: Posttraumatic stress disorder in older adults: a conceptual review. J Anxiety Disord 14:133–156, 2000

Ballard CG, Cassidy G, Bannister C, et al: Prevalence, symptom profile, and aetiology of depression in dementia sufferers. J Affect Disord 29:1–6, 1993

Ballard C, Bannister C, Solis M, et al: The prevalence, associations and symptoms of depression amongst dementia sufferers. J Affect Disord 36:135–144, 1996

Ballard C, Neill D, O'Brien J, et al: Anxiety, depression, psychosis in vascular dementia: prevalence and associations. J Affect Disord 59:97–106, 2000

Ballard C, Johnson M, Piggott M, et al: A positive association between 5HT re-uptake binding sites and depression in dementia with Lewy bodies. J Affect Disord 69:219–223, 2002

Beekman AT, Bremmer MA, Deeg DJ, et al: Anxiety disorders in later life: a report from the Longitudinal Aging Study Amsterdam. Int J Geriatr Psychiatry 13:717–726, 1998

Blazer D, George L, Hughes D: The epidemiology of anxiety disorders: an age comparison, in Anxiety in the Elderly: Treatment and Research. Edited by Salzman C, Lebowitz BD. New York, Springer, 1991, pp 89–96

Blazer DG, Bachar JR, Manton KG: Suicide in late life: review and commentary. J Am Geriatr Soc 34:519–525, 1986

Bohm C, Robinson DS, Gammans RE, et al: Buspirone therapy in anxious elderly patients: a controlled clinical trial. J Clin Psychopharmacol 10:47S–51S, 1990

Bourland SL, Stanley MA, Snyder AG, et al: Quality of life in older adults with generalized anxiety disorder. Aging and Mental Health 4:215–323, 2000

Branconnier RJ, Cole JO, Ghazvinian S, et al: Clinical pharmacology of bupropion and imipramine in elderly depressives. J Clin Psychiatry 44(5 Pt 2):130–133, 1983

Bressler R, Katz MD: Drug therapy for geriatric depression. Drugs Aging 3:195–219, 1993

Burke WJ, Houston MJ, Boust SJ, et al: Use of the Geriatric Depression Scale in dementia of the Alzheimer type. J Am Geriatr Soc 37:856–860, 1989

Burke WJ, Dewan V, Wengel SP, et al: The use of selective serotonin reuptake inhibitors for depression and psychosis complicating dementia. Int J Geriatr Psychiatry 12:519–525, 1997

Burns A, Jacoby R, Levy R: Psychiatric phenomena in Alzheimer's disease, III: disorders of mood. Br J Psychiatry 157:92–94, 1990

Hunt N, Robbins I: The long-term consequences of war: the experience of World War II. Aging and Mental Health 5:183–190, 2001

Hyer L, Summers M, Braswell L, et al: Posttraumatic stress disorder: silent problem among older combat veterans. Psychotherapy 32:348–364, 1995

Jackson CW: Obsessive-compulsive disorder in elderly patients. Drugs and Aging 7:438–448, 1995

Johnston D: A series of cases of dementia presenting with PTSD symptoms in World War II combat veterans. J Am Geriatr Soc 48:70–72, 2000

Kales HC, Blow FC, Copeland LA, et al: Health care utilization by older patients with coexisting depression and dementia. Am J Psychiatry 156:550–556, 1999

Kales HC, Blow FC, Roberts JS, et al: Dementia, depression and coexisting dementia and depression: detection of diagnoses and 12-month health care outcomes (abstract). Am J Geriatr Psychiatry 9:72, 2001

Karel MJ, Hinrichsen G: Treatment of depression in late life: psychotherapeutic interventions. Clin Psychol Rev 20:707–729, 2000

Kathol RG, Noyes R Jr, Williams J, et al: Diagnosing depression in patients with medical illness. Psychosomatics 31:434–440, 1990

Katon W, Schulberg H: Epidemiology of depression in primary care. Gen Hosp Psychiatry 14:237–247, 1992

Katona CL, Aldridge CR: The dexamethasone suppression test and depressive signs in dementia. J Affect Disord 8:83–89, 1985

Katona CL, Hunter BN, Bray J: A double-blind comparison of the efficacy and safety of paroxetine and imipramine in the treatment of depression with dementia. Int J Geriatr Psychiatry 13:100–108, 1998

Katz IR: Diagnosis and treatment of depression in patients with Alzheimer's disease and other dementias. J Clin Psychiatry 59(suppl 9):38–44, 1998

Katz IR, Reynolds CF 3rd, Alexopoulos GS, et al: Venlafaxine ER as a treatment for generalized anxiety disorder in older adults: pooled analysis of five randomized placebo-controlled clinical trials. J Am Geriatr Soc 50:18–25, 2002

Kaufer DI, Cummings JL, Christine D: Effect of tacrine on behavioral symptoms in Alzheimer's disease: an open-label study. J Geriatr Psychiatry Neurol 9:1–6, 1996

Klausner EJ, Alexopoulos GS: The future of psychosocial treatments for elderly patients. Psychiatr Serv 50:1198–1204, 1999

Klerman GL, Weissman MM: Increasing rates of depression. JAMA 261:2229–2235, 1989

Knesevich JW, Martin RL, Berg L, et al: Preliminary report on the affective symptoms in the early stages of senile dementia of the Alzheimer type. Am J Psychiatry 140:233–235, 1983

Koenig HG, Blazer DG: Epidemiology of geriatric affective disorders. Clin Geriatr Med 8:235–251, 1992

Kohn R, Westlake RJ, Rasmussen SA, et al: Clinical features of obsessive-compulsive disorder in elderly patients. Am J Geriatr Psychiatry 5:211–215, 1997

Krasucki C, Howard R, Mann A: The relationship between anxiety disorders and age. Int J Geriatr Psychiatry 13:79–99, 1998

Krystal JH, Leaf PJ, Bruce ML, et al: Effects of age and alcoholism on the prevalence of panic disorder. Acta Psychiatr Scand 85:77–82, 1992

Kunik ME, Braun U, Stanley MA, et al: One session cognitive-behavioural therapy for elderly patients with chronic obstructive pulmonary disease. Psychol Med 31:717–723, 2001

Lazarus LW, Newton N, Cohler B, et al: Frequency and presentation of depressive symptoms in patients with primary degenerative dementia. Am J Psychiatry 144:41–45, 1987

Lebowitz BD, Pearson JL, Schneider LS, et al: Diagnosis and treatment of depression in late-life: consensus statement update. JAMA 278:1186–1190, 1997

Levy ML, Cummings JL, Kahn-Rose R: Neuropsychiatric symptoms and cholinergic therapy for Alzheimer's disease. Gerontology 45(suppl 1):15–22, 1999

Lindesay J: Phobic disorders in the elderly. Br J Psychiatry 159:531–541, 1991

Lindesay J: Phobic disorders and fear of crime in the elderly. Aging and Mental Health 1:81–85, 1997

Lindesay J, Briggs K, Murphy E: The Guy's/Age Concern survey: prevalence rates of cognitive impairment, depression and anxiety in an urban elderly community. Br J Psychiatry 155:317–329, 1989

Lipton M, Schaffer W: Physical symptoms related to post-traumatic stress disorder (PTSD) in an aging population. Military Medicine 153:316–318, 1988

Livingston G, Yard P, Beard A, et al: A nurse-coordinated educational initiative addressing primary care professionals' attitudes to and problem-solving in depression in older people: a pilot study. Int J Geriatr Psychiatry 14:401–405, 2000

Livingston H, Livingston M, Fell S: The Lockerbie disaster: a 3 year follow-up of elderly victims. Int J Geriatr Psychiatry 9:989–994, 1994

Perez-Stable EJ, Miranda J, Munoz RF, et al: Depression in medical outpatients: underrecognition and misdiagnosis. Arch Intern Med 150:1083–1088, 1990

Petracca G, Teson A, Chemerinski E, et al: A double-blind placebo-controlled study of clomipramine in depressed patients with Alzheimer's disease. J Neuropsychiatry Clin Neurosci 8:270–275, 1996

Philip I: DepRelief: training programme for primary care. Int J Clin Psychopharmacol S5:S55–S57, 1998

Port CL, Engdahl B, Frazier P: A longitudinal and retrospective study of PTSD among older prisoners of war. Am J Psychiatry 158:1474–1479, 2001

Radley M, Redston C, Bates F, et al: Effectiveness of group anxiety management with elderly clients of a community psychogeriatric team. Int J Geriatr Psychiatry 12:79–84, 1997

Raj BA, Corvea MH, Dagon EM: The clinical characteristics of panic disorder in the elderly: a retrospective study. J Clin Psychiatry 54:150–155, 1993

Rao V, Lyketsos CG: The benefits and risks of ECT for patients with primary dementia who also suffer from depression. Int J Geriatr Psychiatry 15:729–735, 2000

Rasmussen SA, Eisen JL: The epidemiology and clinical features of obsessive compulsive disorder. Psychiatr Clin North Am 15:743–758, 1992

Reding M, Haycox J, Blass J: Depression in patients referred to a dementia clinic: a three-year prospective study. Arch Neurol 42:894–896, 1985

Regier DA, Farmer ME, Rae DS, et al: One-month prevalence of mental disorders in the United States and sociodemographic characteristics: the Epidemiologic Catchment Area study. Acta Psychiatr Scand 88:35–47, 1993

Reichman WE, Coyne AC: Depressive symptoms in Alzheimer's disease and multi-infarct dementia. J Geriatr Psychiatry Neurol 8:96–99, 1995

Reifler BV, Larson E, Hanley R: Coexistence of cognitive impairment and depression in geriatric outpatients. Am J Psychiatry 139:623–626, 1982

Reifler BV, Teri L, Raskind M, et al: Double-blind trial of imipramine in Alzheimer's disease patients with and without depression. Am J Psychiatry 146:45–49, 1989

Reifler BV: A case of mistaken identity: psuedodementia is really predementia. J Am Geriatr Soc 48:593–594, 2000

Reisberg B, Ferris SH, de Leon MJ, et al: The stage specific temporal course of Alzheimer's disease: functional and behavioral concomitants based upon cross-sectional and longitudinal observation. Prog Clin Biol Res 317:23–41, 1989

Reynolds CF, Frank E, Perel J, et al: Maintenance therapies for late-life recurrent major depression: research and review circa 1995. Int Psychogeriatr 7(suppl):27–40, 1995

Rosen J, Zubenko GS: Emergence of psychosis and depression in the longitudinal evaluation of Alzheimer's disease. Biol Psychiatry 29:224–232, 1991

Rosenthal M, Stelian J, Wagner J, et al: Diogenes syndrome and hoarding in the elderly: case reports. Isr J Psychiatry Relat Sci 36:29–34, 1999

Roth M, Mountjoy CQ, Amrein R: Moclobemide in elderly patients with cognitive decline and depression: an international double-blind, placebo-controlled trial. Br J Psychiatry 168:149–157, 1996

Rovner BW, Ganguli M: Depression and disability associated with impaired vision: the MoVies Project. J Am Geriatr Soc 46:617–619, 1998

Rovner BW, Kafonek S, Filipp L, et al: Prevalence of mental illness in a community nursing home. Am J Psychiatry 143:1446–1449, 1986

Rovner BW, Broadhead J, Spencer M, et al: Depression and Alzheimer's disease. Am J Psychiatry 146:350–353, 1989

Rubin EH, Morris JC, Berg L: The progression of personality changes in senile dementia of the Alzheimer's type. J Am Geriatr Soc 35:721–725, 1987

Sapolsky R: The possibility of neurotoxicity in the hippocampus in major depression: a primer on neuron death. Biol Psychiatry 48:755–765, 2000

Schatzberg AF, Kremer C, Rodriguez HE, et al: Double-blind, randomized comparison of mirtazepine and paroxetine in elderly depressed patients. Am J Geriatr Psychiatry 10:541–500, 2002

Schaub RT, Linden M: Anxiety and anxiety disorders in the old and very old: results from the Berlin Aging Study (BASE) Comprehensive Psychiatry 41(2 suppl 1):48–54, 2000

Schneider LS: Pharmacological considerations in the treatment of late life depression. Am J Geriatr Psychiatry 4(suppl 1):S51–S65, 1996

Schnurr PP, Spiro A III: Combat exposure, posttraumatic stress disorder symptoms, and health behaviors as predictors of self-reported physical health in older veterans. J Nerv Ment Dis 187:353–359, 1999

Schulberg HC, Katon WJ, Simon GE, et al: Best clinical practice: guidelines for managing major depression in primary medical care. J Clin Psychiatry 60(suppl 7):19–26, 1999

Wylie ME, Miller MD, Shear MK, et al: Fluvoxamine pharmacotherapy of anxiety disorders in later life: preliminary open-trial data. J Geriatr Psychiatry Neurol 13:43–48, 2000

Zubenko GS, Moossy J: Major depression in primary dementia: clinical and neuropathologic correlates. Arch Neurol 45:1182–1186, 1988

Zweig RM, Ross CA, Hedreen JC, et al: The neuropathology of aminergic nuclei in Alzheimer's disease. Ann Neurol 24:233–242, 1988

Chapter 2

Dementia

Myron F. Weiner, M.D.

This chapter presents an overview of clinically relevant advances in the diagnosis, treatment, and prevention of dementing illness in older adults. A literal explosion of knowledge about dementing illness in recent years has led to greater accuracy in diagnosis, greater understanding of the pathophysiology of dementing illnesses, greater treatment options, and greater knowledge of risk factors. Strides have been made in the early detection of Alzheimer's disease (AD) and its differentiation from other dementing illnesses. Other advances have led to distinctions between dementing illnesses at a molecular level. New treatments have become available for AD. There have been advances in the prevention of vascular dementia, and based on evidence from epidemiological studies, the possibility of preventive measures for AD is on the horizon.

Diagnosis

The American Academy of Neurology has proposed a set of standards for the evaluation and diagnosis of suspected dementing illness (Knopman et al. 2001). In addition to history-taking, mental status examination, and neurological and general physical examination, the recommendations include screening for depression, assessment of thyroid function, and determination of plasma vitamin B_{12} concentration. Routine screening for syphilis is no longer recommended, but neuroimaging (computed tomography [CT] or magnetic resonance imaging [MRI] scan) is recommended as a routine. The guidelines recommend acceptance of the DSM-IV (American Psychiatric Association 1994) criteria for dementia and the National Institute on Neurological and Communication Disorders and Stroke/Alzheimer's Disease and Related Disorders (NINCDS/ADRDA) criteria (McKhann et al. 1984) for AD. They recommend spinal fluid examination for protein 14–3–3 in cases of suspected Creutzfeldt-Jakob disease, and neuropsychological testing for differentiating frontotemporal dementias from other dementing illnesses.

The use of formal diagnostic criteria is important for research and for planning treatment, but such criteria may also restrict clinicians' vision. For example, NINCDS/ADRDA criteria for AD require that patients be demented. From the standpoint of potential therapies, this may be too late. The pathology of AD is present long before individuals become so cognitively impaired that they meet criteria for dementia; waiting to treat the disease until individuals become frankly demented is much like waiting to treat hypertension until after patients suffer their first stroke. For this reason, clinical investigators are searching for the earliest signs suggesting the future development of full-blown AD, and a proposal has been made to establish a diagnostic category of mild cognitive impairment (MCI).

Mild Cognitive Impairment

Small decrements in learning and retrieval are part of normal aging. Some individuals develop more severe memory deficits that appear stable, whereas others go on to develop AD or other dementing illnesses. To categorize those with "benign" memory loss, a syndrome of age-associated memory impairment (AAMI) was proposed by Crook et al. (1986). Criteria for AAMI include complaints of gradual memory loss in persons of older than 50, objective evidence of impairment on a standardized memory test (as compared with the mean established for young adults), evidence of adequate intellectual function, and absence of dementia or any medical condition that could produce cognitive deterioration. Although AAMI may be a normal variant of aging, Goldman and Morris (2001) suggested that this may not be so. They followed 202 elderly community-dwelling persons (mean age of 77 years) with and without memory disturbance for an average of 3 years. Among the persons who met "loose" criteria for general cognitive intactness (score on the Short Blessed Test [Blessed et al. 1968] $\leq$ 10), 29% met criteria for AAMI. Of this AAMI group, 42% progressed to dementia over 3 years versus 16% of those initially considered cognitively normal. Among individuals who met a more strict measure of general cognitive normality (Short Blessed Test score $\leq$ 5), 22% of the 202 subjects met AAMI criteria, and progression to dementia occurred in 31% of the AAMI group versus 9% in normal persons.

An effort to detect "preclinical" or prodromal AD has led to the designation of a syndrome of *mild cognitive impairment* (Petersen et al. 1999). Patients with MCI have complaints of abnormal memory and have objective evidence of impaired memory on psychological testing with a verbal memory task, have preserved general cognitive function, and perform their activities of daily living at a normal level. Because the sole detectable cognitive deficit is memory, Petersen et al. (2001a) prefer to term this condition *amnestic MCI*.

A comparison of 76 MCI subjects with 234 healthy control subjects and 106 persons with mild AD showed that subjects with MCI differed cognitively from control subjects only in memory. The groups were similar in memory function to patients with early AD, but differed from early-AD patients in that only one area of cognition (memory) was affected (Petersen et al. 1999). When followed up over 5 years, 10%–15% of these individuals developed AD each year—far in excess of the expected 1%–2% per year expected in the general population. Thus, 50%–80% of the group with MCI met criteria for AD within 5 years of initial diagnosis (Petersen et al. 2001a). Predictors of progression from MCI to AD in this cohort included the presence of an apolipoprotein E ε4 (ApoE ε4) allele, poor performance on a cued recall test, and hippocampal atrophy on MRI.

Morris et al. (2001), using slightly different criteria, compared 177 cognitively normal elders with 277 elders having mild cognitive impairment. The mild impairment group was divided into three subgroups: those who were suspected to be early AD, those thought to be incipient AD, and those with uncertain cause. Over an average of 9.5 years, 100% of the group suspected to be early

AD progressed to dementia. Over 5 years, 61% of the suspected early AD group, 36% of the suspected incipient AD group, and 20% of the uncertain cause group had progressed to dementia, as compared with 6.8% in the cognitively intact group.

If MCI and AAMI represent the earliest stage of AD, should they not be treated as AD? And if so, what would be the most appropriate treatment? Protection against oxidative stress might be a safe, reasonable starting point. Thus, vitamin E at a dosage of 1,000 IU twice daily could be considered, having been found of value in slowing AD progression (Sano et al. 1997). The other standard treatment for AD, the use of a cholinesterase inhibitor, is called into question by the finding of DeKosky et al. (2002). DeKosky's group found no deficit in cortical choline acetyltransferase activity in patients with MCI, but rather, that levels of choline acetyltransferase were elevated in the hippocampus of those with MCI compared with cognitively intact control subjects. This finding suggests that a compensatory mechanism might be in play. On the other hand, cholinesterase inhibitors improve cognitive function in persons with early AD, in whom there is essentially no cholinergic deficit (Davis et al. 1999), and also in cognitively normal adults. It would therefore still be reasonable to treat with cholinesterase inhibitors individuals with troublesome memory problems who are not clinically diagnosable as AD. Although not compensating for a cholinergic deficit, this strategy might give an additional boost to cognitive function. Studies of the use of vitamin E and cholinesterase inhibitors in MCI are now in progress.

Because of the high prevalence of these disorders, and because many affected persons will progress to AD, it seems reasonable to seek inexpensive, low-risk measures with the potential to slow or halt the progression to AD. For example, trials of vitamins B_6, B_{12}, and folic acid are now under way, based on an association between plasma homocysteine concentration, AD, and vascular dementia (Seshadri et al. 2002).

Dementia With Lewy Bodies

With the development of new immunohistochemical staining techniques, it has been found that dementing illnesses associated with Lewy bodies are a common cause of dementia in elders. Lewy bodies are intraneuronal inclusions that contain α-synuclein, phosphorylated neurofilament proteins, ubiquitin, and other substances involved in the elimination of abnormal or damaged proteins (Lowe et al. 1996). Unlike the neurofibrillary tangles of AD, they do not contain the microtubule-associated tau protein. Using stains for ubiquitin, a protein that tags other molecules for degradation, cortical Lewy bodies are found in 20% of persons diagnosed clinically with AD (Perry et al. 1993) and in the 65% of patients with Parkinson's disease (PD) who develop dementia (Mayeux et al. 1992).

Lewy bodies are thought to result from a post-translational modification of α-synuclein that causes fibril formation and aggregation in neurons and glia (Dickson 2001). For that reason, diseases associated with Lewy bodies have come to be termed α-synucleinopathies. Lewy bodies are numerous in the pigmented substantia nigra cells of patients with PD. They occur in small numbers in the cortex in most cases of idiopathic PD (Hughes 1997) and in larger numbers in the neocortex and limbic structures of persons with PD and dementia (Brown et al. 1998). Lewy bodies may be found in the neocortex, limbic structures, and brainstem in association with the neuropathologic features of AD. In these cases, the so-called Lewy body variant of AD (LBV), AD pathology tends to be minimal (Hansen et al. 1990). Lewy bodies also occur in the neocortex, limbic structures, and brain stem (including substantia nigra) in persons with progressive dementing illness without substantial AD pathology; so-called diffuse Lewy body disease (DLBD; McKeith et al. 1996). Lewy body density in the cerebral cortex correlates with severity of cognitive impairment (Haroutunian et al. 2000), suggesting that Lewy bodies may be intimately related to the underlying dementia-causing process. Additionally, they occur in other neurodegenerative disorders such as multiple systems atrophy, progressive supranuclear palsy, and corticobasal degeneration (Lowe et al. 1996).

It is likely that LBV is the confluence of several processes: the β-amyloid and tau pathology associated with the plaques and tangles of AD and the α-synuclein pathology associated with Lewy bodies. The intraneuronal neurofibrillary tangles of AD are composed largely of phosphorylated tau protein that has become dissociated from microtubules (Strong et al. 1995). DLBD, on the other hand, appears to be a pure α-synucleinopathy.

Criteria have been established for the clinical diagnosis of dementia with Lewy bodies (McKeith et al. 1992), but they do not distinguish between LBV and DLBD. These criteria include dementia with fluctuating attention and concentration and at least one of a) visual or auditory hallucinations usually accompanied by delusions, b) mild extrapyramidal symptoms or sensitivity to neuroleptic drugs, or repeated unexplained falls and/or transient clouding or loss of consciousness, and rapid progression to severe dementia. Using these criteria, Hohl et al. (2000) attained on retrospective chart review only 50% diagnostic accuracy (true positive/[true positive + false positive]) for 10 cases diagnosed clinically as dementia with Lewy bodies. More recently, McKeith et al. (1996) modified the criteria to include dementia with at least one of a) fluctuating attention and concentration, b) recurrent well-formed visual hallucinations, c) spontaneous motor features of Parkinsonism. The diagnosis is supported by repeated falls, syncope, transient loss of consciousness, neuroleptic sensitivity, systematized delusions, or hallucinations in other modalities. Using these criteria, and again based on retrospective chart review, diagnostic sensitivity and specificity achieved 0.83 and 0.95 for the presence of cortical Lewy bodies, but no clinical distinction was made between LBV and DLBD (McKeith et al. 2000b).

The essential issue for clinicians, however, is making diagnoses at the time of initial patient evaluation rather than at the end of their course of illness. In such a study, using consensus guidelines for the diagnosis of probable or possible dementia with Lewy bodies, only 4 of the 13 cases in which cortical Lewy bodies were found at autopsy had a premortem diagnosis of dementia associated with Lewy bodies (sensitivity 30.7%, specificity 100%) (Lopez et al. 2002).

Based on these studies and our own clinical experience (Weiner et al. 1996), it is not possible to differentiate with certainty LBV or DLBD from each other or from AD. However, recent imaging studies with positron-emission tomography (PET) and single-photon emission computerized tomography (SPECT) suggest that LBV and DLBD may be differentiated from AD by the presence of reduced glucose uptake or reduced regional cerebral blood flow in the occipital visual association cortex (Okamura et al. 2001).

There is clinical importance to diagnosing dementia with Lewy bodies. Possibly because the cholinergic deficit in LBV is severe (Perry et al. 1994), there may be a good response of behavioral and psychotic symptoms to cholinesterase inhibitors, which are discussed later in this chapter (see "Treatment of Alzheimer's Disease"). There is often neuroleptic sensitivity in patients with dementia with Lewy bodies due to deficits in nigrostriatal dopamine pathways (Barber et al. 2001), making it important in these individuals to use cholinesterase inhibitors or atypical antipsychotics (or both) in the management of psychotic symptoms when they occur.

Frontotemporal Dementias

Frontotemporal dementias (FTDs) are a heterogeneous group of disorders that are less common as a whole than AD or dementias with Lewy bodies. FTDs are slowly progressive, tend to have prominent language or behavioral symptoms, and are often associated with parkinsonism. The best-known FTD is Pick's disease, in which language impairments and behavioral disturbances are associated with focal atrophy of frontal and temporal lobes and microscopic findings of argyrophilic inclusions (Pick bodies) and swollen, achromatic neurons. The three common clinical presentations of FTD are the FTD clinical profile (Neary et al. 1988), primary progressive aphasia (PPA) (Mesulam 2001), and semantic dementia (Hodges et al. 1992). The FTD clinical profile includes executive dysfunction, social and interpersonal conduct problems, and apathy and/or disinhibition. PPA is characterized by expressive aphasia with word-finding difficulty, agrammatism, and phonemic paraphasias. Semantic dementia is a fluent dysphasia with severe difficulty in naming and understanding words and difficulty in stating or demonstrating the function of tools or utensils.

The clinical criteria for FTD overlap considerably with those for AD. In one study, 86% of patients with autopsy-proven Pick's disease were misdiagnosed clinically as having AD (Mendez et al. 1993). New clinical consensus criteria for FTD have been published, but continue to overlap considerably with DSM-IV-TR (American Psychiatric Association 2000) criteria for AD (Table 2–1).

Table 2–1.   Clinical criteria for frontotemporal dementia

---

1. Development of behavioral or cognitive deficits manifested by either
   a. Early and progressive change in personality, with difficulty modulating behavior, often resulting in inappropriate responses or activities or
   b. Early and progressive change in language, characterized by problems with expression of language or severe naming difficulty and problems with word meaning.
2. The deficits in 1a or 1b cause significant impairment in social or occupational function and represent a significant decline from a previous level of function.
3. There is gradual onset and continuing decline of function.
4. The deficits are not due to other nervous system conditions, systemic conditions, or substance use.
5. The deficits do not occur exclusively during a delirium.
6. The diagnosis is not better accounted for by a psychiatric disorder, such as depression.

Source. Adapted from McKhann et al. 2001

Conventional cognitive testing is often insensitive to the early and isolated executive and/or language deficits of patients with FTD. Clinical tests of frontal lobe function include the elicitation of frontal release signs and inability to perform the Luria maneuver. Patients with FTD often display echopraxia, perseveration, and motor impersistence. SPECT imaging, which is used widely in the evaluation of patients with FTD, characteristically shows frontal and temporal perfusion deficits, but no data are available concerning its sensitivity and specificity.

In addition to Pick's disease, PPA, and semantic aphasia, FTDs include frontotemporal degeneration with ubiquitinated inclusions, corticobasal degeneration, progressive supranuclear palsy, and frontotemporal degeneration with neuronal loss and spongiosis. Familial FTD may be due to chromosome 17-linked multiple system tauopathy, whose clinical manifestations include disinhibition, dementia, parkinsonism, and muscle wasting. A frontal type of dementia also occurs in amylotrophic lateral sclerosis; in familial cases, there may be linkage to chromosome 9q21-q22.

Treatment of Frontotemporal Dementias

Because the cholinergic system is not involved in FTD, patients with FTD do not respond to cholinesterase inhibitors. However, selective serotonin reuptake inhibitors (SSRIs) may be useful in treating many of the behavioral symptoms. Other symptomatic treatments that have been tried include dopaminergic therapies for parkinsonism and language problems (Lipton and Weiner 2003).

Alzheimer's Disease

AD is an insidiously progressive degenerative disorder whose prevalence increases until approximately 90 years of age. The full-blown disease is characterized by the triad of amnesia, anomia, and apraxia. There is severe memory impairment accompanied by difficulty naming objects and difficulty initiating and carrying out simple tasks of daily living such as dressing and self-grooming. On average, patients with AD maintain their social skills well into the disease process, at which time behavioral and psychological symptoms may become prominent. These symptoms are largely transient and tend to diminish toward the latter part of the disease, when language is lost and apraxia becomes severe.

The course of AD is often complicated in its latter stages by mild extrapyramidal symptoms. Individuals who live out the entire course of illness become bed-bound and incontinent, unable to verbally express or feed themselves. The terminal event in these cases is usually sepsis due to pneumonia or a urinary tract infection. The course of the illness is from 4 to 20 years. Individuals with presenile-onset illness generally have the most malignant course.

plaques and intraneuronal neurofibrillary tangles. Plaques (except those due to severe head injury) develop over years. They are composed of a central core of beta amyloid, a toxic abnormal degradation product of amyloid precursor protein (APP). So-called mature plaques are surrounded by degenerating neurites and by inflammatory cells. Tangles consist of hyperphosphorylated tau molecules. The relationship between plaques and tangles is unclear, but it has been theorized that the abnormal phosphorylation of tau is related to oxidative stress induced by beta-amyloid toxicity.

Risk Factors

Except for the rare cases of autosomal-dominant AD and in Down's syndrome, the two main risk factors for AD are age and having an affected first-degree relative. Autosomal-dominant AD can result from mutations in one of several genes, including the *APP* gene on chromosome 21, and mutations in the presenilin genes on chromosomes 1 and 14. APP is a long transmembrane protein present in somatic cells. Its function is unknown. The presenilins seem to play a role in brain development. Individuals with Down's syndrome uniformly develop the neuropathology of AD by the fifth decade of life (Wisniewski et al. 1985), probably because persons with Down's syndrome have a reduplication of the *APP* gene that causes an overproduction of amyloid in brain. Other risk factors include head injury with loss of consciousness, inheritance of the ApoE ε4 allele, hypercholesterolemia, and elevated plasma levels of homocysteine.

Head Injury

There appears to be a relationship between severe closed head injury and the subsequent development of AD. The risk is compounded by the inheritance of an ApoE ε4 allele. Mayeux et al. (1995) found a twofold increase in AD among persons with a history of severe head injury when no other known risk factor was present, and a tenfold increase in persons with a history of severe head injury and one or more ApoE ε4 alleles. The mechanism is unknown, but may be related to increased permeability of the blood–brain barrier to toxic substances. Nicoll et al. (1995) reported an association of ApoE ε4 to brain amyloid deposition within weeks following head injury. However, Omeara et al. (1997) found head injury with loss of consciousness to increase risk of AD in men, but not in women, suggesting the possibility of a protective action of estrogen.

Apolipoprotein E ε4 Allele

Apolipoproteins are cholesterol-transporting proteins. In the brain, ApoE, which is synthesized and secreted largely by astrocytes, participates in mobilizing and redistributing lipids in nervous system injury and development (Pitas et al. 1987). ApoE has 3 alleles; 2, 3, and 4. ApoE ε4 is a risk factor for late-onset familial and sporadic AD, presumably by influencing the deposition of beta amyloid in brain (Schmechel et al. 1993). The ApoE ε4 allele occurs in 40% of patients with late-onset AD compared with 14% of the general population. ApoE ε4 allele frequency is increased to 25%–50% in persons with LBV (Weiner et al. 1996), but does not differ from the general population in DLBD (Galasko et al. 1994). The normal ApoE ε4 allele frequency in DLBD suggests that AD and DLBD differ in pathogenesis. Although there is no way to change the inheritance of ApoE ε4, it is possible that means may be found to reduce the expression of this carrier molecule, for example, by reducing plasma cholesterol concentration.

Hypercholesterolemia

Elevated plasma cholesterol appears to be an independent risk factor for AD (Notkola et al. 1998) and may be related to enhancement of amyloid deposition by cholesterol. Cholesterol depletion, on the other hand, inhibits the generation of beta amyloid in neurons (Simons et al. 1998). The finding that a statin drug lowers brain production of cholesterol (Locatelli et al. 2002) may indicate the mechanism by which this class of drugs may have a preventive effect (see "Drugs and Hormones" later in this chapter).

Hyperhomocysteinemia

High plasma homocysteine levels (above 14 mmol/L) have been associated with increased risk for the development of AD. An analysis of data from the Framingham study showed a twofold increase in risk for developing AD over 8 years (Seshadri et al. 2002). There are many potential pathways for homocysteine toxicity, including increased oxidative stress and potential excitotoxic damage to neurons. Because hyperhomocysteinemia is potentially reversible by treatment with vitamins B_6, B_{12}, and folic acid, this is a promising avenue for potential prophylaxis against AD or for slowing of AD progression.

Protective Factors

Retrospective reviews of a number of databases have yielded important clues with regard to possible protective agents and lifestyle considerations. These, of course, do not establish causal relationships. In the case of drugs and hormones, they may reflect quality of overall self-care.

Drugs and Hormones

Many retrospective studies suggest a protective effect in AD for estrogen (LeBlanc et al. 2001), nonsteroidal anti-inflammatory drugs (NSAIDs; in 't Veld et al. 2001), and statin drugs (Jick et al. 2000). Protective effects may require at least 2 years' exposure to NSAIDs (in't Veld et al. 2001), but the dosage needed is not clear. These putative protective effects need to be confirmed by prospective studies.

The data are most convincing for the statin drugs. A 70% reduction in risk for AD was found in a large retrospective study (Jick et al. 2000). A comparable reduction was found in another study in subjects younger than 80 years of age even after adjustment for sex, educational level, and self-rated health (Rockwood et al. 2002). This is especially hopeful because this class of drugs can be prescribed for both women and men and poses less danger than either estrogen (deep vein thrombosis, stimulation of estrogen-dependent malignancies) or NSAIDs (gastrointestinal bleeding).

Education/Mental Activity

Does level of educational attainment, intelligence, or intellectual activity level prevent AD or mitigate the course of the disease?

These questions have given rise to a large body of literature in relation to prevalence, incidence, and course of AD (Weiner et al. 1998). The subject is important because these issues are commonly raised by families in their attempts to help loved ones and to institute preventive measures for themselves. Families almost always want to know how much effort to expend in engaging affected family members in "mind-building" activities.

With regard to prevalence, the findings are unclear. They are based on the assumption that most elderly persons who developed dementia had AD. For example, Katzman et al. (1988) found that in subjects over 75 years of age, the relative risk of developing dementia was twice as great for subjects with no education as for those with elementary or middle school education. However, Fratiglioni et al. (1993) found no association between level of education and dementia prevalence. Dementia incidence was also unaffected by education in the Framingham study (Cobb et al. 1995). Another prospective study found the risk of dementia to be twice as great in persons with low education (5.3 ± 2.6 years) and low occupation levels as in subjects with high education (13.0 ± 2.8 years) and high occupation levels. In this study, 101 of the 106 persons who became demented met clinical criteria for AD (Stern et al. 1994).

Do better-educated persons have greater cognitive reserve? This possibility is supported by an inverse relationship that was found between level of education, level of occupational achievement, and regional cerebral blood flow in persons with AD (Stern et al. 1992, 1995b). This suggested that bright or high-achieving persons did not manifest the disease clinically until more extensive tissue damage had been done. In addition, Alexander et al. (1997) found that estimates of premorbid intellectual ability correlated inversely with regional cortical metabolism. On the other hand, Teri et al. (1995) found that AD patients with higher education declined 1.2 Mini-Mental State Examination points per year more than those with a less-than–high school education; persons with 13 or more years of education declined 1.3 points per year more rapidly. Similarly, Edland et al. (1993) found that for every 4 years of education, subjects had a 0.6 point per year more rapid decline on Mini-Mental State Examination score.

Reports of a relationship between education and length of survival with AD are also in conflict. When Stern et al. (1995a) compared survival of AD patients whose educational level was less than 8 years with those whose level was more than 8 years, they found decreased survival in the more educated group. By contrast, Heyman et al. (1996) found that in a large registry, the only significant predictors of survival were age, sex, and severity of dementia.

Moritz and Petitti (1993) found in a large sample of persons with AD that in those with less education, age of onset was significantly later and impairment was greater, whereas duration of illness was not significantly different. Weiner et al. (1998) found in two large databases that higher education was associated with earlier reported onset of AD symptoms. There was a slightly earlier reported onset of AD symptoms in more educated persons and no difference in time between initial evaluation and death between groups with higher (> 11 years) or lower (< 11 years) levels of education.

In summary, it seems unlikely that education or intelligence strongly influence the incidence, prevalence, or clinical course of AD. Of greater immediate importance is the issue of mental stimulation. Do high levels of intellectual stimulation reduce the risk of AD? Friedland et al. (2001) found that greater time devoted to intellectual, passive, and physical activities from early adulthood to middle adulthood was associated with a significant decrease in risk for developing AD. In a prospective study, a group of Catholic nuns, priests, and brothers were followed annually for up to 7 years (Wilson et al. 2002). Baseline scores were obtained for frequency of participation in common cognitive activities, such as reading a newspaper. Those individuals reporting greater intellectual activity at baseline had significantly reduced decline in global cognition, working memory, and perceptual speed. Reports such as these are often taken by caregivers of patients with AD to mean that attempting to keep their loved ones cognitively stimulated may mitigate the progression of the disease. The authors of the studies recognize, by contrast, that the differences in intellectual and other activities may well represent the earliest manifestations of the disease. After all, the pathology of AD develops silently over years before the threshold of dementia is crossed.

In the light of these findings, what do we tell our patients and their families? A reasonable position is that no strong evidence has yet shown that efforts at intellectual problem solving are a prophylactic against or affect the onset or course of AD. Based on this, an appropriate course of action would be to encourage patients with AD and their family members to engage in those activities they find comfortable, but as a source of interest or pleasure rather than to improve or prolong their cognitive function.

Treatment

The treatments presently available for AD are directed toward ameliorating processes that occur toward the end of a pathophysiologic cascade that presumably begins with the abnormal processing of APP and ends in neuronal death. Drugs augmenting the cholinergic system are used to compensate for loss of cholinergic neurons' input to the neocortex. Antioxidants are used to reduce the toxic byproducts of the inflammation induced by beta amyloid deposits in the brain.

Drugs Acting on the Cholinergic System

The use of these drugs is based in part on the fact that AD is a disease of memory and that the cholinergic system is important for the encoding of memory. It is known that small doses of a cholinesterase inhibitor improve memory in normal persons and that anticholinergic agents impair cognition in normal persons. Furthermore, the effects of anticholinergic agents are reversed by cholinesterase inhibitors. In AD, there is profound loss of neocortical cholinergic innervation principally due to depopulation of the nucleus basalis of Meynert (Whitehouse et al. 1982). These findings have provided the basis for attempting to enhance central cholinergic function in AD. The most successful attempts have employed cholinesterase inhibitors. Acetylcholine precursors and agonists have not been useful, and the latter have frequently had adverse effects.

worsening as compared with 42% of the placebo group (Rogers et al. 1998). On a measure of global function, approximately 25% of the donepezil-treated group (5 or 10 mg) improved, compared with 11% of the placebo group. If administered at bedtime, donepezil may produce disturbing, vivid dreams. The medication is available in 5 and 10 mg tablets, with slightly greater efficacy at 10 mg daily. Donepezil's low affinity for CYP2D6 and 3A4 makes drug–drug interactions unlikely.

Rivastigmine has a half-life of approximately 2 hours. It is converted to an inactive metabolite at the site of action and is not metabolized by the liver (Jann 2000). The effective dose of rivastigmine is 6–12 mg/day administered in divided doses twice daily with food, but many individuals are unable to tolerate 12 mg/day. Rivastigmine is available in tablets of 1.5, 3, 4.5, and 6 mg.

Galantamine, in addition to its cholinesterase inhibition, modulates the response of nicotinic receptors to acetylcholine. Galantamine is well absorbed and has a terminal elimination half-life of 7 hours. The drug is metabolized by the hepatic P450 isoenzymes and by glucuronidation and is also excreted unchanged in the urine. Effective doses of galantamine are 24 and 32 mg/day (Raskind et al. 2000), administered twice daily in divided doses. It is available in 4-, 6-, and 8-mg tablets.

Cholinesterase inhibitors are used with caution in persons with complete heart block, sinus bradycardia, and in the presence of active peptic ulcer disease or asthma. Drug–drug interactions are uncommon. Patients and their families need to be counseled about the concomitant use of highly anticholinergic drugs such as amitriptyline, imipramine, diphenhydramine, and oxybutynin.

It is difficult to know when these drugs should be withdrawn. I generally continue them until the family is no longer able to manage the patient at home. When a patient is admitted to a long-term care facility, I begin a slow downward titration. If there is considerable worsening of function, I generally increase the dose or restart the drug. Other clinicians maintain these medications as long as individuals maintain the ability to interact socially.

Cholinesterase Inhibitors for Behavioral and Psychological Symptoms of Alzheimer's Disease

Many behavioral/emotional symptoms in AD may be related to cholinergic deficit and might therefore respond to cholinergic treatment. Cummings (2000) postulated that behavioral and psychological symptoms in AD might be due to loss of input from cholinergic neurons in the basal forebrain to the limbic and paralimbic regions and to the cerebral cortex. In support of this hypothesis, Cummings et al. (2000) found that over a period of 6 months, donepezil-treated patients (as compared with unmedicated patients) were significantly less likely to be threatening, destroy property, or talk loudly, and fewer were receiving sedatives. In a 12-month study, Weiner et al. (2000) found that donepezil treatment modestly improved depressive symptoms and behavioral dysregulation.

In a placebo-controlled study evaluating a cholinesterase inhibitor (rivastigmine) for the treatment of emotional/behavioral symptoms in persons diagnosed clinically with dementia with Lewy bodies, 120 subjects were enrolled for a study that lasted 20 weeks. Most of the completers in this study (92%) were able to tolerate a total dose of 6 mg/day. There was no change in extrapyramidal symptoms or in Mini-Mental State Examination or Clinical Global Change scores, but patients receiving rivastigmine were significantly less anxious and apathetic and had fewer delusions and hallucinations than control subjects, based on observed cases (McKeith et al. 2000a).

Based on controlled studies, the case for the use of cholinesterase inhibitors for treatment emotional/behavioral symptoms in persons with AD or suspected dementia with Lewy bodies is not strong. However, many clinicians, including myself, have had the experience that treating patients who have prominent hallucinations and mild extrapyramidal symptoms with cholinesterase inhibitors often dramatically reduces the psychotic symptoms.

Antioxidants

Based on the hypothesis that free radical damage might contribute to the progression of AD, Sano et al. (1997) conducted a 2-year

vaccine can be made is a question that remains to be answered because inflammation would seem a predictable consequence of creating an antigen-antibody reaction in brain.

Interrupting Tangle Formation. As mentioned earlier, neurofibrillary tangle formation is the result of the hyperphosphorylation of the microtubule-associated protein tau. Formation of tangles may interrupt transportation of molecule with neurons and thus interfere with their metabolism and their ability to remodel or make synaptic connections and may ultimately cause cell death. Tau is phosphorylated by glycogen synthase kinase-3β (GSK-3beta) and is inhibited via protein kinase C. Of interest, lithium has been shown to block tau hyperphosphorylation by inhibition of GSK-3beta (Lovestone et al. 1999); thus, inhibitors of GSK-3beta such as lithium and valproic acid may be future therapeutic agents for AD.

Treatment of Behavioral Symptoms

Patients with AD can experience the entire range of severe psychopathology, from psychosis to mood disturbance, although mania is quite rare. Suicide is also a rare event. Psychotic symptoms seen in patients include the delusion that their homes are not their homes or that their spouses are planning to desert or abandon them. Another symptom is visual hallucinations, sometimes threatening, and sometimes merely puzzling—such as seeing strange children running in and out of the house. Major depression is rare (Weiner and Doody 2002), but loss of initiative and loss of interest are common. Patients frequently become upset when challenged with tasks beyond their abilities, but they usually recover quickly when distracted.

Many types of behavior disturbance appear in the middle stage of AD that seem unrelated to psychosis or mood disturbance. These patients frequently "shadow" their caregivers, becoming frightened when caregivers are out of sight, and are often unable to tolerate the tension of being left outside the door while caregivers are using the toilet. Middle-stage patients often become disturbed when their routine is interrupted and as they fail to recognize familiar faces and surroundings.

Some of the behaviors seen are related to disinhibition, such as fondling other nursing home residents. Overt aggression occurs when disinhibition is compounded by irritability. Patients may strike caregivers who are trying to rush them into a shower or bath. Indeed, refusal to bathe is a common behavioral problem that is not well understood. Management of these behaviors in late-stage AD is dealt with at length in Mahoney et al. (2000).

At this time, there is no satisfactory single approach that family caregivers can employ in dealing with their loved ones' behavioral symptoms. At best, family caregivers can be aided in helping their loved ones find a "comfort zone" in which they can operate. For example, many patients with AD do well in a structured daily routine in their home environment but develop behavioral symptoms when removed from that routine and context, as, for example, an infrequent visit to church or to the home of a relative. In these cases, caregivers are asked to allow their loved ones to remain in their routines at home, including supporting them in activities that individual patients may value highly, such as writing checks or gardening, and supporting them with unobtrusive cues.

Formal behavioral programs administered by family caregivers have not been successful for moderate to severe behavioral disturbances (Teri et al. 2000), but the use of psychotropic drugs had little better success. Many psychotropic drugs have been found to have off-label use in the treatment of behaviorally disturbed patients with AD. These largely include antipsychotic agents with minimal anticholinergic effects because anxiolytic agents increase confusion and lead to falls and because anticholinergic drugs also add to confusion. The use of psychotropic drugs for behavioral symptoms in AD has been reviewed extensively by Weiner and Schneider (2003).

A few simple principles govern the use of psychotropic drugs for behavioral disturbances. These include obtaining information about the interpersonal and environmental context in which the behaviors arose—with whom, under what circumstances, where, and how often. Patients' physical condition needs to be assessed because behavioral symptoms can result from injury, pain, infec-

tion, and a host of other physical causes. When behaviors constitute an ongoing danger to patients or caregivers, whether in
terms of direct harm or physical and emotional exhaustion, psychotropic agents should be administered on a daily basis and
continued at the effective dose until the behaviors have been adequately controlled for some time. After a reasonable interval,
which may be weeks or months, attempts can be made to reduce
the dose or to discontinue the medication. The aim, in this in-
stance, is to prevent the behaviors from recurring. Unlike the
symptoms of psychotic illnesses such as schizophrenia or mood
disturbances such major depression, behavioral symptoms tend
to be transient; thus, it is rarely necessary to continue psychotropic drugs for more than 6 months. On the other hand, when
behavioral symptoms occur rarely, it is appropriate to use as-
needed psychotropic medications.

Many behaviors, such as wandering, rummaging, and pacing,
do not respond to behavioral or psychopharmacologic measures.
They are dealt with by having patients maintained in an environment that tolerates these behaviors. Incontinence is dealt with by
prompted toileting until patients no longer respond to prompting. When prompting fails, incontinence pads are indicated.
Sleep–wake disturbances are best dealt with prophylactically, by
keeping patients alert and active during the day. This exhausts
many caregivers and may be feasible only in the setting of long-
term care.

Vascular Dementia

Vascular dementia accounts for about 15% of late-life dementing
illness and is associated with the signs and symptoms of cerebrovascular disease. Dementia rarely occurs in the absence of one
or more frank strokes. Vascular dementia is considered when
cognitive symptoms follow one or more strokes within 3 months,
when there is a stair-step pattern of decline, and when there are
localizing or lateralizing neurological signs or symptoms. The
presence of strokes can usually be confirmed by structural brain
imaging procedures such as CT scan or MRI. Many persons experience a combination of AD and one or more strokes.

Treatment

The course of individual strokes is often one of acute deficit followed by full or partial recovery of function, depending on the size and location of the stroke. Efforts may be made acutely to limit the extent of tissue death in thrombotic stroke by the use of thrombolytic agents. Rehabilitative efforts include physical and speech therapy, as appropriate, as part of a comprehensive restorative program. The long-term treatment of vascular dementia consists basically of preventing further strokes, which are usually thrombotic and usually the result of atherosclerosis.

Vasodilators

Vasodilators are ineffective in cerebrovascular insufficiency because they reduce perfusion pressure throughout the brain and shunting blood from areas of high resistance.

Antiplatelet Agents

Platelet antiaggregants such as aspirin, ticlopidine (Ticlid), and clopidogrel reduce transient ischemic attacks and thrombotic strokes. Aspirin commonly causes gastric irritation and gastrointestinal bleeding and rare instances, causes thrombocytopenia. Employing an enterically coated 81-mg preparation reduces the gastrointestinal complications. Ticlopidine is more effective than aspirin (Hass et al. 1989), and its chief side effects are diarrhea and skin rash. An uncommon side effect is severe reversible neutropenia, which occurs within the first 3 months of treatment. It is dosed at 250 mg twice daily.

Clopidogrel has approximately the same efficacy as aspirin in reducing the combined risk of thrombotic stroke, myocardial infarction, or vascular death (Jarvis and Simpson 2000). Drug interactions are rare, but this drug may cause severe thrombocytopenia. Gastrointestinal hemorrhage was slightly less frequent with this drug than aspirin. It causes occasional diarrhea or skin rash but is unlikely to cause neutropenia. The dosage is 75 mg once a day.

Dipyridamole (Persantine) is a platelet adhesion inhibitor. A large clinical trial of persons who had experienced a transient ischemic attack or stroke were randomized to placebo, aspirin (50 mg once daily), sustained-release dipyridamole (400 mg once daily), or a combination of aspirin and dipydridamole (Forbes 1998). Dipyridamole and aspirin reduced the recurrence of stroke by 16% and 18%, respectively, as compared with placebo. Combination of the drugs resulted in a 37% reduction in stroke recurrence as compared with placebo. Dipyridamole is administered in doses ranging from 25–100 mg four times daily.

Prevention

Prevention includes prophylaxis of transient ichemic attacks, examination of extracranial vessels for surgically correctable stenosis, control of hypertension and diabetes, reduction of serum cholesterol when appropriate, and anticoagulation in the case of atrial fibrillation.

Hypolipidemic Agents

Drugs that inhibit the enzyme 3β-hydroxy-3β-methylglutaryl-coenzyme A (HMGCOA) reductase (so-called statin drugs) block hepatic synthesis of cholesterol and significantly reduce cardiovascular events, including stroke. It has been recommended that persons with established atherosclerosis be treated with a statin to achieve a low-density lipoprotein cholesterol level less than 100 mg/dL (Ansell 2000).

Hyperhomocysteine-Lowering Agents

Epidemiologic studies have shown hyperhomocysteinemia (plasma concentration > 12 micromoles/L) to be associated with increased risk for atherosclerotic cardiovascular disease (Herrmann 2001). Research is now underway to determine the impact of reducing homocysteine levels in blood using high-dose folic acid and B vitamins.

Cognitive Rehabilitation/Memory Training

A considerable body of literature has arisen on the use of non-pharmacologic techniques to enhance the cognitive abilities and reduce the disabilities of persons with various forms of brain damage (reviewed in Cicerone et al. 2000). Cognitive rehabilitation is a group of techniques that encompasses memory training, among others. Cognitive rehabilitation is a part of most programs for the rehabilitation of persons with traumatic brain injury (TBI). It is defined as a systematic, functionally oriented service of therapeutic activities based on assessment and understanding of individuals' brain-behavioral deficits. Interventions include reinforcing or reestablishing previously learned behavior patterns, establishing new cognitive activity patterns through compensatory mechanisms for impaired brain systems, establishing new activity patterns through external compensatory mechanisms (like reminder notebooks) or environmental structuring and support, and enabling persons to adapt to their cognitive disability. These interventions may address attention, concentration, perception, memory, comprehension, communication, reasoning, problem solving, judgment, initiation, planning, and self-monitoring. In addition to TBI, cognitive rehabilitation techniques are employed in stroke rehabilitation, and they have more recently been applied to neurodegenerative disorders such as AD.

It is difficult to assess these techniques because they are individualized and then applied collectively, based on the cognitive profile presented by patients. Despite the need, there has been considerable resistance to conducting placebo-controlled studies in the setting of rehabilitation from acute TBI, despite the fact that many of the therapeutic techniques have not been objectively validated in randomized controlled trials. Essentially the only randomized trial in the setting of acute TBI was carried out in young adults.

Salazar (2000) studied 120 active-duty military personnel who had sustained moderate-to-severe closed head injuries. They were assigned randomly to an intensive, standardized 8-week in-hospital cognitive rehabilitation program or a limited home rehabilitation program with weekly telephone support from a psychiatric nurse. At 1-year follow-up no difference was found in the primary outcome measure (return to work); 90% or more returned to work from both groups. There were also no differences in cognitive, behavioral, or quality-of-life measures in this group of healthy young men. It is probably not reasonable to generalize the results of this study to older adults with multiple medical problems.

Cognitive rehabilitation has also been employed with individuals with more remote TBI. In a randomized, controlled clinical trial, outreach treatment (average of two sessions per week for approximately 27 weeks) in participants' homes, day centers, or workplace was compared with provision of written literature detailing alternative resources. Subjects had experienced TBI from 3 months to 20 years previously. At 2-year follow-up, 48 outreach and 46 information participants were assessed. Those who had received the outreach intervention were significantly more likely to have made gains in functional status (regardless of length of time since injury) but not in productive employment, socialization, anxiety, or depression (Powell et al. 2002).

Cognitive rehabilitation has also been attempted in persons with AD. Quayhagen et al. (1995) compared active cognitive stimulation with passive cognitive stimulation and a wait-list control group in persons with AD. Families in the treatment group had 12 weekly in-home training sessions that included both caregivers and patients. Following this, cognitive interventions were administered by caregivers for 60 minutes each day for 12 weeks. The interventions addressed memory, problem solving, and social interaction. Patients in the treatment condition improved in general cognitive function, memory, and verbal fluency by the end of the 12-week intervention but declined to baseline after 9 months. The placebo group remained static and the control group declined below baseline. The outcome of this study is similar to the outcome with cholinesterase inhibitors, but the intensity of the training required and the amount of effort required of caregivers seems quite impractical.

We have compared the effects of treatment with the cholinesterase inhibitor donepezil alone with donepezil plus a program of cognitive-linguistic stimulation on cognitive and linguistic function and quality of life in persons with mild to moderate AD. Individuals being treated with donepezil were randomized to a treatment (donepezil plus cognitive-linguistic stimulation) or control condition (donepezil). Patients and caregivers were assessed at baseline, 6 months, and 1 year. The cognitive-linguistic stimulation program included 10 individual sessions with patients and 2 sessions with caregivers to instruct them in maintaining cognitive-linguistic stimulation at home. The intervention sessions were followed by bimonthly contacts consisting of two sessions, one to provide intervention and one to provide caregiver support. At 1 year, there was no difference between groups in cognitive test scores, language use, functional status, or quality of life measures (Chapman TB, Weiner MF, Zleutz J, unpublished data, 2003).

Importantly, the findings from studies of cognitive enrichment programs do not support the "use it or lose it" concept in relation to AD. Cognitive enrichment programs appear to raise or maintain morale in certain individuals, but persons with AD appear to lose ground at an equal rate regardless of the richness of their cognitive input or strivings. An unfortunate side effect of efforts by caregivers to improve cognition by these measures is that caregivers often experience mounting guilt over not having done enough to help sustain their loved ones.

Memory retraining has been employed with persons with AAMI with modest success. Older adults with memory complaints who were followed up 3 years after participation in a self-taught memory program showed no long-term effect (Scogin and Bienias 1988). Persons with static cognitive deficits due to acute episodes such as stroke, head trauma, or central nervous system infection appear to profit from memory training, but there are essentially no controlled studies. These patients also can be helped to recognize the need to pace themselves slowly, to stay with what is familiar, and to use external reminders.

Management of behavioral symptoms is based on the same general principles observed for patients with AD.

Summary

The enormous strides made in recent years in the diagnosis, treatment, and prevention of dementing illness are encouraging signs of what the near future may hold in store. Further progress will require continued interaction between clinical observation, clinical laboratory testing, and basic laboratory science. Clinicians, epidemiologists, population geneticists, biochemists, and molecular biologists all have further contributions to make. We look to clinicians to establish more refined diagnostic categories and to carry out clinical trials. We look to epidemiologists to uncover risk and protective factors. We look to geneticists to uncover the genes responsible for disease phenotypes, and we look to laboratory scientists to determine the biochemical and molecular roots of neurodegenerative disease and to point to areas of potential therapeutic intervention.

We have come a long way since the time when dementia was thought to be a normal consequence of old age and, more recently, of "hardening of the arteries," but we still have a very long way to go in maximizing the potential of our fellow humans.

References

Aisen PS, Davis KL, Berg JD, et al: A randomized controlled trial of prednisone in Alzheimer's disease. Alzheimer's Disease Cooperative Study. Neurology 54:588–593, 2000

Alexander GE, Furey ML, Grady CL, et al: Association of premorbid intellectual function with cerebral metabolism in Alzheimer's disease: implications for the cognitive reserve hypothesis. Am J Psychiatry 154:165–172, 1997

American Psychiatric Association: Diagnostic and Statistical Manual of Mental Disorders, 4th Edition. Washington, DC, American Psychiatric Association, 1994

American Psychiatric Association: Diagnostic and Statistical Manual of Mental Disorders, 4th Edition Text Revision. Washington, DC, American Psychiatric Association, 2000

Ansell BJ: Cholesterol, stroke risk, and stroke prevention. Curr Atheroscler Rep 2:92–96, 2000

Anthony JC, Breitner JC, Zandi PP, et al: Reduced prevalence of AD in users of NSAIDs and H2 receptor antagonists: the Cache County study. Neurology 54:2066–2071, 2000

Barber R, Panikkar A, McKeith IG: Dementia with Lewy bodies: diagnosis and management. J Geriatr Psychiatry 16(suppl 1):S12–S18, 2001

Blessed G, Tomlinson BE, Roth M: The association between quantitative measures of dementia and of senile change in the cerebral gray matter of elderly subjects. Br J Psychiatry 114:797–811, 1968

Brown DF, Dababo MA, Bigio EH, et al: Neuropathologic evidence that the Lewy body variant of Alzheimer disease represents coexistence of Alzheimer disease and idiopathic Parkinson disease. J Neuropathol Exp Neurol 57:39–46, 1998

Cicerone KD, Dahlberg C, Kalmar K, et al: Evidence-based cognitive rehabilitation: recommendations for clinical practice. Arch Phys Med Rehabil 81:1596–1615, 2000

Cobb JL, Wolf PA, Au R, et al: The effect of education on the incidence of dementia and Alzheimer's disease in the Framingham study. Neurology 45:1707–1712, 1995

Crook T, Bartus RT, Ferris SH, et al: Age-associated memory impairment. Proposed diagnostic criteria and measures of clinical change: report of a National Institute of Mental Health Work Group. Devel Neuropsychol 2:261–276, 1986

Cummings JL: Cholinesterase inhibitors: a new class of psychotropic compounds. Am J Psychiatry 157:4–15, 2000

Cummings JL, Donohue JA, Brooks RL: The relationship between donepezil and behavioral disturbances in patients with Alzheimer's disease. Am J Geriatr Psychiatry 8:134–140, 2000

Davis KL, Samuels SJ: Advances in the treatment of Alzheimer's disease, in The Dementias: Diagnosis, Treatment, and Research, 3rd Edition. Edited by Weiner MF, Lipton AM. Washington, DC, American Psychiatric Publishing, 2003

Davis KL, Mohs RC, Marin D, et al: Cholinergic markers in elderly patients with early signs of Alzheimer disease. JAMA 281:1401–1406, 1999

DeKosky ST, Iknonomovic MD, Styren SD, et al: Upregulation of choline acetyltransferease activity in hippocampus and frontal cortex of elderly subjects with mild cognitive impairment. Ann Neurol 51:145–155, 2002

Dickson DW: Alpha-synuclein and the Lewy body disorders. Curr Opin Neurol 14:423–432, 2001

Edland SD, Clark CM, Kukull WA: Relationship of education to change in MMSE score: a CERAD finding. Gerontologist 33:207–208, 1993

Forbes CD: Secondary stroke prevention with low-dose aspirin, sustained release dipyridamole alone and in combination. Thromb Res 92(suppl 1):S1–S6, 1998

Fratiglioni L, Ahlbohm A, Viitanen M, et al: Risk factors for late-onset Alzheimer's disease: a population-based case-control study. Ann Neurol 33:258–266, 1993

Friedland RP, Fritsch T, Smyth KA, et al: Patients with Alzheimer's disease have reduced activities in midlife compared with healthy control-group members. Proc Natl Acad Sci U S A 98:3440–3445, 2001

Galasko D, Hansen L, Katzman R, et al: Clinical-neuropathological correlations in Alzheimer's disease and related dementias. Arch Neurol 51:888–895, 1994

Goldman WP, Morris JC: Evidence that age-associated memory impairment is not a normal variant of aging. Alzheimer Dis Assoc Disord 15:72–79, 2001

Hansen L, Salmon D, Galasko D, et al: The Lewy body variant of Alzheimer's disease: a clinical and pathological entity. Neurology 40:1–8, 1990

Haroutunian V, Serby M, Purohit DP, et al: Contribution of Lewy body inclusions to dementia in patients with and without Alzheimer disease neuropathological conditions. Arch Neurol 57:1145–1150, 2000

Hass WK, Easton JD, Adams HP Jr: A randomized trial comparing ticlopidine hydrochloride with aspirin for the prevention of strokes in high-risk patients. N Engl J Med 321:501–507, 1989

Herrmann W: The importance of hyperhomocysteinemia as a risk factor for diseases: an overview. Clin Chem Lab Med 39:666–674, 2001

Heyman A, Peterson B, Fillenbaum G, et al: The Consortium to Establish a Registry for Alzheimer's disease (CERAD), part XIV: demographic and clinical predictors of survival in patients with Alzheimer's disease. Neurology 46:656–660, 1996

Hodges JR, Patterson K, Oxbury S, et al: Semantic dementia: progressive fluent aphasia with temporal lobe atrophy. Brain 115:1783–1806, 1992

Hohl U, Tiraboschi P, Hansen LA, et al: Diagnostic accuracy of dementia with Lewy bodies. Arch Neurol 57:347–351, 2000

Hughes AJ: Clinicopathologic aspects of Parkinson's disease. Eur Neurol 38(suppl 2):13–20, 1997

in 't Veld BA, Ruitenberg A, Hofman A, et al: Nonsteroidal antiinflammatory drugs and the risk of Alzheimer's disease. N Engl J Med 345:1515–1521, 2001

Jann MW: Rivastigmine, a new-generation cholinesterase inhibitor for the treatment of Alzheimer's disease. Pharmacotherapy 20:1–12, 2000

Janus C, Pearson J, McLaurin J, et al: A beta peptide immunization reduces behavioural impairment and plaques in a model of Alzheimer's disease. Nature 408:979–82, 2000

Jarvis B, Simpson K: Clopidogrel: a review of its use in the prevention of atherothrombosis. Drugs 60:347–377, 2000

Jick H, Zornberg GL Jick SS, et al: Statins and the risk of dementia. Lancet 356:1627–1631, 2000

Katzman R, Zhang M, Qu W-Y, et al: A Chinese version of the Mini-Mental State Examination: impact of illiteracy in a Shanghai dementia survey. J Clin Epidemiol 41:971–978, 1988

Knopman DS, DeKosky ST, Cummings JL, et al: Practice parameter: diagnosis of dementia (an evidence-based review). Neurology 56:1143–1153, 2001

LeBlanc ES, Janowsky J, Chan BK, et al: Hormone replacement therapy and cognition: systematic review and meta-analysis. JAMA 285:1489–1499, 2001

Lipton AM, Weiner MF: Differential diagnosis, in The Dementias: Diagnosis, Treatment, and Research, 3rd Edition. Edited by Weiner MF, Lipton AM. Washington, DC, American Psychiatric Publishing, 2003

Locatelli S, Lutjohann D, Schmidt HH-J, et al: Reduction of plasma 24S-hydroxycholesterol (cerebrosterol) levels using high-dosage simvastatin in patients with hypercholesterolemia. Arch Neurol 59:213–126, 2002

Lopez OL, Becker JT, Kaufer DI, et al: Research evaluation and prospective diagnosis of dementia with Lewy bodies. Arch Neurol 59:43–46, 2002

Lovestone S, Davis DR, Webster MT, et al: Lithium reduces tau phosphorylation: effects in living cells and in neurons at therapeutic concentrations. Biol Psychiatry 45:995–1003, 1999

Lowe JS, Mayer RJ, Landon M: Pathological significance of Lewy bodies in dementia, in Dementia With Lewy Bodies. Edited by Perry R, McKeith I, Perry E. Cambridge, UK, Cambridge University Press, 1996, pp 21–32

Mahoney EK, Volicer L, Hurley AC: Management of Challenging Behaviors in Dementia. Baltimore, MD, Health Professions Press, 2000

Mayeux R, Denero J, Hemenigildo N, et al: A population-based investigation of Parkinson's disease with and without dementia: relationship to age and gender. Arch Neurol 49:492–497, 1992

Mayeux R, Ottman R, Maestre G, et al: Synergistic effects of traumatic head injury and apolipoprotein-E ε4 in patients with Alzheimer's disease. Neurology 45:555–557, 1995

McKeith IG, Perry RH, Fairbairn AF, et al: Operational criteria for senile dementia of Lewy body type (SDLT). Psychol Med 22:911–922, 1992

McKeith IG, Galasko D, Kosaka K, et al: Consensus guidelines for the clinical and pathological diagnosis of dementia with Lewy bodies (DLBD): Report of the consortium on DLBD international workshop. Neurology 47:1113–1124, 1996

McKeith IG, Del Ser T, Spano P, et al: Efficacy of rivastigmine in dementia with Lewy bodies: a randomized, double-blind, placebo-controlled international study. Lancet 16:2031–2036, 2000a

McKeith IG, Ballard CG, Perry RH, et al: Prospective validation of consensus criteria for the diagnosis of dementia with Lewy bodies. Neurology 54:1050–1058, 2000b

McKhann G, Drachman D, Folstein M, et al: Clinical diagnosis of Alzheimer's disease: report of the NINCDS-ADRDA work group under the auspices of the Department of Health and Human Services Task Force on Alzheimer's disease. Neurology 34:939–944, 1984

McKhann GM, Albert MS, Grossman M, et al: Clinical and pathological diagnosis of frontotemporal dementia. Arch Neurol 58:1803–1809, 2001

Mendez MF, Selwood A, Mastri AR, et al: Pick's disease versus Alzheimer's disease: a comparison of clinical characteristics. Neurology 43:289–292, 1993

Mesulam M-M: Primary progressive aphasia. Ann Neurol 49:425–432, 2001

Moritz DJ, Petitti DB: Association of education with reported age of onset and severity of Alzheimer's disease at presentation: implications for use of clinical samples. Am J Epidemiol 137:456–462, 1993

Morris JC, Storandt M, Miller JP, et al: Mild cognitive impairment represents early stage Alzheimer disease. Arch Neurol 58:397–405, 2001

Mulnard RA, Cotman CW, Kawas C, et al: Estrogen replacement therapy for treatment of mild to moderate Alzheimer disease: a randomized controlled trial. Alzheimer's Disease Cooperative Study. JAMA 283:1007–1015, 2000

Neary D, Snowden JS, Northen B, et al: Dementia of frontal lobe type. J Neurol Neurosurg Psychiatry 51:353–361, 1988

Nicoll JAR, Roberts GW, Graham DI: Apolipoprotein E ε4 allele is associated with deposition of amyloid β-protein following head injury. Nature Med 1:135–137, 1995

Notkola IL, Sulkava R, Pekkanen J, et al: Total serum cholesterol, apolipoprotein E epsilon 4 allele, and Alzheimer's disease. Neuroepidemiol 17:14–20, 1998

Okamura N, Arai H, Higuchi M, et al: [18F] FDG-PET study in dementia with Lewy bodies and Alzheimer's disease. Prog Neuropsychopharmacol Biol Psychiatry 25:447–456, 2001

Omeara ES, Kukull WA, Sheppard L, et al: Head injury and risk of Alzheimer's disease by apolipoprotein E genotype. Am J Epidemiol 146:373–384, 1997

Peterson RC, Smith GE, Waring SC, et al: Mild cognitive impairment: clinical characterization and outcome. Arch Neurol 56:303–308, 1999

Petersen RC, Doody R, Kurz A, et al: Current Concepts in Mild Cognitive Impairment. Arch Neurol 58: 1985–1992, 2001a

Petersen RC, Stevens JC, Ganguli M, et al: Practice parameter. Early detection of dementia: mild cognitive impairment (an evidence-based review). Neurology 56:1133–1142, 2001b

Perry EK, Irving DI, Kerwin JM, et al: Cholinergic transmitter and neurotrophic activities in Lewy body dementia: similarity to Parkinson's and distinction from Alzheimer's disease. Alz Dis Assoc Disord 7:69–79, 1993

Perry EK, Haroutunian V, Davis KL, et al: Neocortical cholinergic activities differentiate Lewy body dementia from classical Alzheimer's disease. Neuroreport 21:747–749, 1994

Pitas RE, Boyles JK, Lee SH, et al: Astrocytes synthesize apolipoprotein E and metabolize apolipoprotein E-containing lipoproteins. Biochim Biophys Acta 917:148–161, 1987

Powell J, Heslin J, Greenwood R: Community based rehabilitation after severe traumatic brain injury: a randomized controlled trial. J Neurol Neurosurg Psychiatry 72:193–202, 2002

Quayhagen MP, Quayhagen M, Corbeil RR, et al: A dyadic remediation program for care recipients with dementia. Nurs Res 44:153–159, 1995

Raskind MA, Peskind ER, Wessel T, et al: Galantamine in AD: a 6-month randomized, placebo-controlled trial with a 6-month extension. Neurology 54:2261–2268, 2000

Rockwood K, Kirkland S, Hogan DB, et al: Use of lipid-lowering agents, indication bias, and the risk of dementia in community-dwelling elderly people. Arch Neurol 59:223–227, 2002

Rogers J, Kirby LC, Hempelman SR, et al: Clinical trial of indomethacin in Alzheimer's disease. Neurology 43:1609–1611, 1993

Rogers SL, Farlow MR, Doody RP, et al: A 24-week, double-blind, placebo-controlled trial of donepezil in patients with Alzheimer's disease. Neurology 50:136–145, 1998

Salazar AM, Warden DL, Pehwab K, et al: Cognitive rehabilitation for traumatic brain injury: a randomized trial. JAMA 283:3075–3081, 2000

Sano M, Ernesto C, Thomas RG, et al: A controlled trial of selegiline, alpha-tocopherol, or both as treatment for Alzheimer's disease. N Engl J Med 336:1216–1222, 1997

Chapter 3

Late-Life Psychoses

George T. Grossberg, M.D.
Abhilash K. Desai, M.D.

Introduction

Psychoses are serious psychiatric disorders because of their clinical significance and social impact. Delusions and hallucinations are the hallmarks of psychotic disorders, although catatonic behavior as well as bizarre behaviors may also be evidence of impaired reality testing. Almost any type of psychosis that occurs in younger persons can be seen in older patients. Psychotic symptoms cause substantial psychosocial morbidity, frequently affecting patients' relationships with spouses or partners, children, and other family members as well as their ability to care for themselves and other aspects of their lives. A thorough understanding of these disorders is crucial to ensuring a successful outcome.

Prevalence of Psychotic Disorders in the Elderly

The prevalence of psychotic disorders in the elderly ranges from 0.2%–5.7% in community-based samples to 10% in a nursing home population (Christenson and Blazer 1984; Henderson and Kay 1997; Henderson et al. 1998). A more recent study found an even higher prevalence (10%) of psychotic symptoms in nondemented individuals aged 85 and older (Ostling and Skoog 2002). There is an increased incidence of psychotic symptoms in elderly patients in contrast to younger adults (Thorpe 1997). In the United States, there are currently over 4 million cases of Alzheimer's disease (AD), and it is estimated that this number will exceed 14 million by the year 2050 (Brookmeyer and Gray 2000). More than 50% of patients with AD have some form of psychosis at some point during the course of their illness (Paulsen et al. 2000). Approximately 2% of the population over age 54—about 1 million persons—have chronic mental illness other than dementia (Gurland and Cross 1982). Older persons with schizophrenia make up the majority of these patients. The number and proportion of older adults with schizophrenia is expected to more than double in the next three decades (Palmer et al. 1999). In patients over 65 years of age, prevalence rates of bipolar disorder range from 0.1% to 0.4%. In addition, 5%–12% of geriatric psychiatry admissions are for bipolar disorder (Leuchter and Spar 1985). Late-onset psychoses account for about 10% of the psychiatric admissions of older adults (Van Gerpen et al. 1999). As the population ages, the absolute number of elderly individuals developing psychotic symptoms will rise dramatically.

Risk Factors Associated With Psychosis in the Elderly

A number of potential risk factors may predispose the elderly to developing psychotic symptoms (Christenson and Blazer 1984; Grossberg and Manepalli 1995; Henderson and Kay 1997; Henderson et al. 1998; Ostling and Skoog 2002; Van Gerpen et al. 1999). These include comorbid psychiatric illnesses (especially dementia and delirium), genetic predisposition, female gender, social isolation, sensory deficits (visual and hearing impairment), cognitive changes, polypharmacy, certain premorbid personality traits (cold and querulous, schizotypal, paranoid), poor caretaker relationships, bedridden condition, early life trauma, and substance abuse. Association with sensory deficits may be due, at least in part, to a suboptimal correction of sensory deficits in older psychiatric patients. Social isolation could also reflect premorbid traits or adaptive response to having psychotic symptoms. Addressing risk factors (e.g., correction of visual deficits or hearing impairment) in management will improve treatment outcomes.

Classification of Psychotic Disorders in the Elderly

Psychotic disorders can be classified as follows (see Table 3–1):

- *Primary psychotic disorders*: Includes schizophrenia and related disorders, bipolar disorder, unipolar psychotic depression, delusional disorder.
- *Secondary psychotic disorders*: Includes delirium with psychotic features, psychoses associated with dementia, and psychotic symptoms secondary to an identifiable medical condition or chemical agent (prescribed and over-the-counter medications, street drugs, and alcohol).
- *Comorbid psychotic disorder (two psychotic disorders occurring in the same individual)*: Examples include, but are not limited to, patients with schizophrenia and psychoses related to alcohol use disorder, affective psychoses comorbid with psychosis due to a chemical agent, dementia with psychoses and superimposed delirium, and psychoses associated with delirium in patients with primary psychotic disorders.

Psychotic disorders in old age have more toxic (e.g., drugs), metabolic (e.g., laboratory abnormalities), and structural (e.g., brain lesions, tumors) associations and a greater association with dementia (Soares and Gershon 1997). Older patients may develop psychotic symptoms as a result of an unrecognized, potentially treatable medical disease. Failure to identify secondary psychotic disorders may result in inappropriate administration of antipsychotics that may further obscure underlying medical conditions causing the psychotic symptoms. Certain secondary psychotic disorders (such as delirium and psychosis due to a general medical condition), if not recognized and treated promptly, can be fatal. Patients with secondary psychotic disorders are at higher risk of serious adverse effects such as extrapyramidal symptoms (EPS) and tardive dyskinesia (TD) with conventional antipsychotics compared with those with primary psychotic disorders. Many secondary psychotic disorders are iatrogenic, that is, they are caused by a failure to recognize the cor-

Table 3–1. Classification of psychotic disorders in the elderly

A) Primary psychotic disorders
   Schizophrenia and related disorders
      Schizophrenia
      Schizoaffective disorder
      Schizophreniform disorder
      Delusional disorder
      Brief psychotic disorder
   Affective psychoses
      Bipolar disorder with psychotic features
      Unipolar depression with psychotic features
B) Secondary psychotic disorders:
   Psychotic symptoms associated with dementia
      Alzheimer's disease with psychoses
      Vascular dementia with psychoses
      Lewy body disease with psychoses
      Other dementing disorders with psychoses
   Psychotic symptoms during delirium
   Psychotic symptoms associated with medications and substance
      abuse
   Psychotic symptoms due to medical and surgical disorders

rect diagnosis or by administration of inappropriate medications such as anticholinergics, especially to patients with dementia. Appropriate therapeutic choices may decrease the incidence of late-onset psychoses (Webster and Grossberg 1998).

Comorbidity

Medical illness may precipitate psychiatric decompensation, delay psychiatric intervention, and have a positive impact on psychiatric outcome when treated successfully. Psychiatric comorbidity may lead to noncompliance of treatment for medical conditions. Also, medical comorbidity is underappreciated and underdiagnosed in older persons with schizophrenia and other psychiatric disorders. Inadequate psychiatric care in long-term care facilities may result in the development of dementia going unrecognized in patients with schizophrenia (Targum and Abbott 1990). The overall prevalence rate of concurrent mental and substance use disorders among older psychiatric patients in a nonacute, public residential psychiatric treatment facility was 21% (Speer and Bates 1992). Alcoholism is prevalent among schizophrenic persons of all age groups and older persons with major depression. Psychosis in the elderly may contribute to nonadherence of antipsychotics as well as nonpsychiatric medications (e.g., antihypertensives, antidiabetic agents). Cardiovascular and pulmonary mortality among patients with untreated bipolar disorder is also high. Early recognition of comorbid medical and psychiatric disorders may decrease serious complications, such as hospitalization.

Approach to an Elderly Patient With Psychotic Symptoms

The diagnosis of psychosis among the elderly requires comprehensive evaluation (Figures 3–1 and 3–2). A thorough history is critical. History is obtained from the patient and at least one significant other familiar with the patient. For patients who are socially isolated, information from neighbors, home health workers, or staff from state agencies who assist the patient should be sought. The physician should also ask about a family history of psychiatric illness (e.g., mood disorder, suicide, schizophrenia, dementia). Consultation with family members and significant others may be extremely useful in establishing family history and identifying prior psychotic or affective episodes. A thorough review of prescription and over-the-counter medications is recommended. Alcohol and illicit drug use should be sought. Once drug toxicity and substance use disorders have been ruled out, either a structural brain lesion such as a tumor or stroke or a subtle seizure disorder such as temporal lobe dysfunction should be considered. "First-rank" symptoms of schizophrenia can occur in psychoses accompanying diagnosable brain disease (Feinstein and Ron 1990). Neuroimaging should be considered in all elderly with late onset of psychotic symptoms and no obviously identifiable etiology. It should also be considered in patients with primary psychotic disorders with an atypical presentation or patients whose illness is resistant to standard pharmacotherapy.

Primary Psychotic Disorders

Schizophrenia

Most elderly with schizophrenia have a long history of psychiatric symptoms (referred to as early onset schizophrenia [EOS]). Approximately 15% have late-onset schizophrenia (LOS), in which onset of symptoms occurs after age 44 (Howard et al. 2000). LOS has also been called middle-age-onset schizophrenia (Palmer et al. 2001). Cases occurring after age 60 can be termed "very-late-onset schizophrenia-like psychosis" (Howard et al. 2000).

Schizophrenia in older persons is among the most expensive disorders when total costs are considered on a per-person basis. It should be considered in the differential diagnosis of all elderly patients with chronic (more than 6 months) psychotic symptoms. The presence of delusions and hallucinations are the hallmark of this disorder. Up to 40% of older persons with schizophrenia may develop clinical depression. Depressive symptoms are associated with worse functioning in older patients with schizophrenia. Typically, persons with EOS experience bizarre delusions (e.g., a stranger has removed his or her organs and replaced them with someone else's organs) that have a predominantly persecutory theme. Auditory hallucinations are the second most prominent psychotic symptom. Schneiderian first-rank symptoms, such as thought broadcasting or two voices arguing with each other, may be present. Patients with EOS may also exhibit formal thought disorder (such as loosening of association), inappropriateness of affect, catatonic symptoms, and negative symptoms.

LOS is generally similar to EOS in terms of positive symptoms (delusions and hallucinations), family history, and chronicity of the course of the disorder (Jeste et al. 1997). However, LOS differs from EOS in several aspects. LOS is more common in women than men, is typically of the paranoid type, and is characterized by better premorbid adjustment and a requirement for lower doses of antipsychotic medications than EOS (Jeste et al. 1997). Also, LOS is associated with a lower prevalence of negative symptoms (social withdrawal, emotional blunting), inappropriateness of affect, and formal thought disorder compared with

EOS (Jeste et al. 1997). Patients with LOS have better neurop chological performance (particularly in learning and abstract/ cognitive flexibility) and possibly larger thalamic volume compared with patients with EOS (Palmer et al. 2001). Aging is associated with complete remission in social deficits in over one-quarter of those with EOS, while another 40% show a marked improvement in symptoms, especially positive symptoms, although in many patients negative symptoms may increase (Belitsky and McGlashan 1993; Ciompi 1980).

Visual hallucinations have correctly been taken as suggestive of toxic/metabolic/structural abnormalities, especially if auditory hallucinations are absent, but it must be recalled that visual hallucinations are common in idiopathic schizophrenia. Neurological examination of older adults with schizophrenia appears to be significantly more abnormal than that of healthy comparison subjects and clinical abnormalities appear to correlate more strongly with age and cognitive impairment than with psychopathology.

Older persons with EOS may exhibit neuropsychological deficits early in the disorder, and because of aging and other lifetime deprivations (e.g., lower education and lower employment, institutionalization), their cognitive functioning may further decline into later life. Usually these deficits are neither as severe nor as progressive as in Alzheimer's disease (Heaton et al. 2001; Palmer et al. 2001). However, a high rate of non-Alzheimer's dementia and accelerated rate of cognitive decline in institutionalized elderly with schizophrenia has also been reported (Harvey et al. 1999). Elderly patients with schizophrenia are more likely to be single and socially isolated. Delusions in schizophrenia are complex and well systematized compared with simple delusions in dementia patients. The schizophrenic patient may have a disturbance in language production but relative paucity of neologisms (compared with an aphasic patient); excellent comprehension, lack of significant cognitive loss, and lack of altered consciousness will usually readily identify the schizophrenic patient from patients with aphasia, dementia, or delirium. The possibility of older persons with schizophrenia developing late-life dementia should be kept in mind.

usually elicits at least one previous episode of affective disorder (which may or may not have been treated).

Psychoses Associated With Bipolar Disorder

Psychotic symptoms (e.g., delusions, hallucinations) are commonly seen during episodes of mania or depression but are more common in the former, appearing in over one-half of manic episodes. Catatonic features may develop in up to one-third of patients during a manic episode. Psychotic symptoms may be mood congruent or mood incongruent. Although most patients with bipolar disorder (BD) have their first episode in their younger days, onset as late as in the ninth and tenth decades has been reported (Umapathy et al. 2000). Late-onset BD (onset after age 50) is more likely to have psychotic features, be associated with a lower rate of familial illness than early onset cases, and have greater medical and neurologic comorbidity. Late-onset BD may also have longer episode durations or more frequent episodes of illness. Of individuals with onset of mania in later life, one-half have had previous depressive episodes, often with a long latency period before the first manic episode. Some cases of mania may be etiologically related to medical diseases, medications used to treat those diseases, and substance use. Cerebrovascular disease, especially right-sided lesions, have been implicated in late-onset mania. Because manic states in the elderly probably represent various disorders with multiple biological determinants, no single characterization of "mania" can be considered to be prototypic. Elderly manic patients are rarely euphoric and more commonly present with irritability, paranoia, or mild confusion (Targum and Abbott 1990). The mortality rate for elderly patients with BD seems to be greater than the community base rate for this age group and also appears to exceed that of geriatric depression patients. Patients with bipolar disorder are at high risk for suicide.

Treatment.   All patients with late-onset manic symptoms should be evaluated carefully for general medical and neurological causes. General principles of treating BD patients with psychoses are similar to those for younger adults. Older patients will usually require lower doses of medications. BD with mania and psychoses can be treated with mood stabilizers alone (lithium, valproate) or with the addition of an atypical antipsychotic agent (such as risperidone, olanzapine or quetiapine). Many elderly patients tolerate only low serum levels of lithium (e.g., 0.4–0.6 mEq/L) and can respond to these levels. Conventional antipsychotics are effective in acute mania but may exacerbate postmanic depression. Electroconvulsive therapy may be useful, especially for catatonic patients with BD, patients whose BD is refractory to psychotropics, and BD patients with psychotic depression. A small number of older patients within the double-blind trials of olanzapine (mean modal dose, 16 mg/day) in patients with bipolar mania demonstrated improvement in mania (Street et al. 2000a). Clozapine is reserved for use in refractory cases.

Psychotic Unipolar Depression

Major depressive disorder may be accompanied by hallucinations or delusions; these may be congruent or noncongruent with the depressive mood. Unipolar depression in later life is often of a psychotic or delusional nature. Psychotic depression occurs in 20%–45% of hospitalized elderly depressed patients (Meyers 1992). Elderly depressed patients have a higher percentage of cognitive symptoms such as disorientation, memory loss, and distractibility, making differentiation from dementia difficult at times. Late-onset depression has been associated with ventricular enlargement, white matter hyperintensities, and cortical atrophy. The delusions are usually mood congruent, with a hopeless content expressed, and may include perceptions of persecution, guilt, suspiciousness, immorality, and somatic delusions. Hallucinations may also occur and can sometimes include commands pertaining to suicide. Depressive delusions can be distinguished from the delusions of dementia patients in that the latter are less systematized and less congruent with the affective disturbance. Psychotic depressive patients have more pronounced agitation or retardation. The presence of delusions appears to run true through repeated episodes. A higher morbidity risk for depression has been reported in the families of psychotic depressive patients than in nonpsychotic depressive patients. In contrast to nonpsychotic depression, elderly patients with psychotic depression are at increased risk for relapse and have more persistent symptoms (e.g., lasting more than 1 year), suicide, hospitalizations, comorbidity, and financial dependency (Flint and Rifat 1998).

Treatment. Major depressive disorder with psychotic features responds better to treatment with a combination of an antipsychotic and an antidepressant than to treatment with either agent alone. Some data indicate that older adults with psychotic depression may respond less well to combination of antidepressant and antipsychotic (Meyers 1998). Continuation treatment of delusional depression in older adults with a conventional antipsychotic and antidepressant does not decrease relapse rates but may be associated with significant untoward adverse events (EPS, TDs, and falls) after recovery from a delusional depression (Meyers et al. 2001). Hence, atypical antipsychotics are preferred over conventional antipsychotics. Electroconvulsive therapy is highly effective in major depressive disorder with psychotic features and at times may be considered a first-line treatment for this disorder.

Schizoaffective Disorder

If a patient has significant mood and psychotic symptoms for 6 or more months, and there is at least a 2-week period of psychotic symptoms in the absence of mood symptoms, schizoaffective disorder should be considered. DSM-IV-TR (American Psychiatric Association 2000) indicates that young adults with schizoaffective disorder will more likely have a bipolar type, whereas older adults more commonly will have a depressive type.

Delusional Disorder

The essential feature of delusional disorder is the presence of one or more nonbizarre delusions (i.e., delusions involving situations that may occur in real life, such as being poisoned, having a disease, or experiencing spousal infidelity) that persist for at least

1 month. Auditory or visual hallucinations, if present, are not prominent. These patients are often single women who live alone and are socially isolated; they not uncommonly have auditory or visual deficits (Targum and Abbott 1990). Tactile or olfactory hallucinations may be present (and prominent) if they are related to the delusional theme (e.g., the sensation of being infested with insects associated with delusions of infestation, or the perception that one emits a foul odor from a body orifice associated with delusion of reference). Apart from the direct impact of the delusions, psychosocial functioning is not markedly impaired, and behavior is neither obviously odd nor bizarre. Mood symptoms, if present, occur briefly compared with the total duration of the delusional periods. DSM-IV mentions that delusional disorder tends to have an age of onset in middle or late adult life. Typically, the patient has been experiencing symptoms for months to years before their illness is identified and treated. Delusions of persecution, delusions of reference, and delusions of infidelity are typical, although somatic delusions and delusions of infestation (also called delusional parasitosis) are not uncommon. Patients with delusional parasitosis have an unshakable belief that they are infested with parasites. Most cases in the literature involve delusions of parasites in the skin. Delusional disorder may be of "mixed type" when more than one type of nonbizarre delusions are present.

Treatment

Atypical antipsychotic drugs are often efficacious, especially in agitated delusional patients. Some patients may be refractory to antipsychotic therapy. One common problem in the treatment of patients with delusional disorder is noncompliance. Supportive psychotherapy is an important modality of treatment for this disorder.

Other Psychotic Disorders

Brief psychotic disorder (formerly known as reactive psychotic disorder) involves psychotic symptoms of less than 1 month in duration usually after a severe stressor. Schizophreniform disorder is diagnosed when a patient meets all criteria for schizophrenia except duration, which is less than 6 months but more than 1 month. Shared psychotic disorder is used when a close relationship with a person (or persons) with an already-present delusion results in the new development of a similar delusion in the second person. Posttraumatic stress disorder (PTSD) may manifest with vivid symptoms of reliving past trauma that may closely mimic auditory and visual hallucinations. It should be considered in the differential diagnosis of psychoses in vulnerable patient groups (e.g., elderly veterans or war survivors, elderly victims of domestic abuse).

Secondary Psychotic Disorders

Psychotic Symptoms Associated With Dementing Disorders

Late-life dementias are associated not only with deficits in cognition and self-care but also with noncognitive psychiatric and behavioral symptoms, including psychosis. Psychosis, characterized by delusions and hallucinations, develops in more than one-third of patients and is one of the most serious complications of dementia. The most common delusions associated with dementing disorders are of people stealing, breaking in, or having intentions to persecute the patient or of food being poisoned. Often the delusional ideas in dementia have an ad hoc quality: a purse is misplaced, and the delusion arises that someone is stealing personal items. Delusions, consisting largely of misconceptions or misidentifications, are common. Common beliefs or behaviors include mistaken suspicion of marital infidelity, beliefs that other patients or caregivers are trying to hurt the patient, fear of personal harm or theft, the belief that the patient's house is not his or her home, misidentification of others (or of the patient's own mirror reflection), and the belief that characters on television are real. With increasing cognitive impairment, the complexity of delusions is reduced. Many patients with dementia experience visual agnosia, in which they do not recognize a person or believe that they are someone else. Hallucinations are also found in these patients. Visual hallucinations are most common, followed by auditory hallucinations or combined auditory and visual hallucinating experiences. Typical visual hallucination content includes persons from the past (such as deceased parents), intruders, animals, complex scenes, or inanimate objects. Most auditory hallucinations seen in patients with dementia tend to be simple kind (hearing dead spouses and other relatives) rather than persecutory ones, although the latter sometimes occur. Capgras' syndrome and reduplicative paramnesia are particularly common with Alzheimer's dementia and Lewy body dementia (LBD). Visual hallucinations may be indicative of a co-occurring delirium. When delusions or hallucinations occur in a patient with dementia, the clinician must first exclude a supervening toxic-metabolic encephalopathy. Psychotic symptoms in patients with dementia are a common trigger for verbal and/or physical aggression. The most common cause for institutionalization in patients with dementia is not severity of memory problems but severity of behavioral problems, including psychosis. Psychotic symptoms in these patients are also responsible for considerable caregiver distress.

Treatment

Mild psychotic symptoms associated with dementia are best managed with nonpharmacological interventions and cholinesterase inhibitors. If antipsychotics are used, the goals should be modest (reduction of emotional distress and behavioral disturbances) compared with a more aggressive goal of remission in affective psychoses. A dose decrease or discontinuation is recommended periodically for all patients with psychoses associated with dementia who receive antipsychotic medications (Alexopoulous et al. 1998). Although conventional or typical neuroleptics are somewhat better than placebo for dementia patients with psychosis (Schneider et al. 1990), the effect is modest and the high risk of toxicity (especially EPS and TD) usually makes them inappropriate. The major predictor of relapse in the same study (Schneider et al. 1990) was agitated and aggressive features. Even low-potency conventional antipsychotics are associated with high frequency of EPS in patients with dementia. Risperidone has the largest body of currently available evidence among the atypical antipsychotics for the treatment of psychoses associated with dementia. Two 12-week, double-blind, placebo-controlled trials of risperidone (1 mg was found to be the optimal dose) included nearly 1,000 test subjects with dementia (AD, vascular dementia, and related disorders) (DeDyn et al. 1999; Katz et al. 1999). Doses of 0.5–1.5 mg/day do not have significantly increased incidence of side effects, but nonetheless are effective in controlling psychosis-driven behavioral disturbances and aggression. Risperidone was superior to haloperidol in terms of efficacy, while presenting a significantly more benign side effect profile. Risperidone at doses higher than 1.5 mg is associated with increased EPS, although in some patients with dementia, EPS can occur even at lower dosages. Risperidone is effective and well tolerated over 13–46 months for nursing home residents with dementia and behavioral disturbances, despite high rates of medical comorbidity and use of concomitant medications (Goldberg 1999). A 6-week, double-blind, placebo-controlled study of olanzapine was conducted in 206 nursing home patients with AD or vascular dementia plus psychosis or severe agitation (Street et al. 2000b). Patients received either placebo or olanzapine 5 mg, 10 mg, or 15 mg. The most effective doses turned out to be 5 mg or 10 mg. The 15-mg dose was not better than placebo but produced significant gait disturbance and sedation. In some patients with dementia, gait disturbance can occur even at lower dosages. A large, multicenter, open-label study of quetiapine found it to be useful for psychotic symptoms in the elderly, many of whom had dementia (McManus et al. 1999). The average daily dose was about 100 mg. Another study found quetiapine beneficial over 52 weeks in dementia patients with psychosis (Tariot et al. 2000). Elderly patients with dementia who are receiving conventional antipsychotics should be switched to atypical antipsychotics to minimize risk of EPS and TD. Cholinesterase inhibitors may benefit mild psychotic symptoms in dementia patients (Cummings 2000). A recent study found the antidepressant citalopram to be more efficacious than placebo in the short-term hospital treatment of psychotic symptoms and behavioral disturbances in nondepressed patients with dementia (Pollock et al. 2002).

Psychoses Associated With Alzheimer's Disease

Delusions and hallucinations are common in AD, with a prevalence of 30%–40%. In a recent study, the cumulative incidence of hallucinations and delusions was 20.1% at 1 year, 36.15% at 2 years, 49.5% at 3 years, and 51.3% at 4 years (Paulsen et al. 2000). AD patients with EPS (parkinsonian gait, bradyphrenia) have twice the frequency of psychosis compared with AD patients without EPS. The presence of psychotic symptoms in patients with AD may identify a distinct phenotype. AD with psychosis is associated with more severe cognitive deficits, more rapid functional and cognitive decline, and premature institutionalization (Farber et al. 2000).

Numerous biological determinants for psychosis in AD have recently been identified (Holroyd et al. 2000; Mega et al. 2000; Sultzer 1996; Sweet et al. 1998, 2001). They include but are not limited to the following: a selective increase in a subtype of striatal dopamine receptor D3; dopamine receptor genetic polymorphisms; specific neuropsychological deficits, specifically frontal or executive function deficits; reduced perfusion in several brain regions, notably the prefrontal cortex, the left striatum, and the left parietal cortex; and atrophy of the right medial temporal lobe and occipital lobe. Patients with AD who have a sibling with AD and psychosis were found to be more than twice as likely to also have psychotic behaviors (Sweet et al. 2002). Impaired visual acuity and severity of cognitive impairment may be associated with visual hallucinations in patients with AD. Glasses and cataract surgery need evaluation as prophylactic or adjunctive treatments for visual hallucinations in patients with probable AD. Psychotic disorder in AD can be reliably diagnosed when patients present with delusions and/or hallucinations that are persistent or episodic for at least 1 month, that are disabling, and that cannot be accounted for by delirium, drugs, or another disorder. The psychosis of AD tends to wax and wane more than that of schizophrenia. A significant number of patients with AD also develop transient psychotic symptoms that remit spontaneously or with cholinesterase therapy.

Psychoses Associated With Vascular Dementia

Vascular dementia, formerly called multi-infarct dementia, may be associated with paranoid psychotic features with a prevalence ranging from 9% to 40% (Cummings et al. 1987). Complex delusions are more characteristic of vascular dementia than AD. Hallucinations are commonly visual and may underlie delusions. Most patients have a history of significant cerebrovascular disease (multiple strokes) and multiple risk factors (e.g., diabetes mellitus, hypertension) accompanying cognitive impairment. T2-weighted magnetic resonance imaging scans are superior to computed tomography in depicting vascular lesions in the brain, which may be subtle. Classically, vascular dementia is characterized by a sudden onset of illness and a stepwise decline in cognitive function rather than the insidious onset and gradually progressive course of AD. Focal neurological signs also point toward vascular dementia. Most patients in the community who have vascular dementia also have AD (Neuropathology Group of the Medical Research Council Cognitive Function and Ageing Study 2001). Vascular dementia without AD accounts for probably only 5% of dementia cases. Emerging data indicate that persons with vascular dementia also benefit from cholinesterase inhibitors.

Psychoses Associated With Lewy Body Disease

LBD is probably the second most common form of degenerative dementia, accounting for up to 20% of cases in the elderly. It is characterized by fluctuating cognitive impairment, spontaneous parkinsonism, and recurrent visual hallucinations. Visual hallucinations early in the course of dementia should alert the clinician to the possibility of LBD. Parkinsonian manifestations are usually mild and do not respond well to dopamimetic agents. Fluctuating cognitive impairment is quite dramatic. Impairment in cognitive reaction time and attention and fluctuation of attentional impairments are more marked in patients with LBD than in patients with AD and may help differentiate the two in the early stages of dementia (Ballard et al. 2001). Patients with LBD are very sensitive to even microdoses of antipsychotics such as haloperidol and may become rigid and immobile even after one or two doses. Accurate diagnosis of LBD as a cause of psychotic symptoms is clinically important in view of the high incidence (60%) of adverse and life-threatening reactions to conventional antipsychotics. The only double-blind, placebo-controlled study in patients with LBD found rivastigmine to be significantly better than placebo in improving behavioral disturbances and psychotic symptoms (McKeith et al. 2000). Case reports of donepezil have also found it to be beneficial in LBD. Cholinesterase inhibitors should be considered as drugs of first choice before instituting antipsychotic medications for treating psychotic symptoms in patients with LBD. If antipsychotic medication is required, atypical antipsychotics with the least likelihood of dose-dependent EPS, such as quetiapine, should be considered, and high-potency atypicals such as risperidone should be avoided.

Psychosis Associated With Frontotemporal Dementias

Frontotemporal dementia (FTDs) are a group of degenerative dementias that are less common than AD, vascular dementia, or LBD and are frequently misdiagnosed. FTDs may account for up to 25% of presenile dementia (dementia before the age of 65). Language impairment (decreased speech output and verbal stereotypes), personality changes (especially apathy), and behavioral disturbances (disinhibition, hyperorality, ritualistic compulsive behaviors) are prominent features from the earliest stages. Patients with FTD have more euphoria, aberrant motor activity, and disinhibition and significantly fewer delusions compared with patients with AD or LBD (Hirono et al. 1999). Bizarre and grandiose delusions are more common with FTD and vascular disease, reflecting loss of frontal lobe monitoring of thought. They may not respond well to cholinesterase inhibitors and for moderate to severe psychotic symptoms, atypical antipsychotics should be considered.

Psychotic Symptoms Accompanying Delirium

Delirium is an acute confusional state characterized by fluctuating levels of consciousness and may be accompanied by illusions, visual hallucinations, and delusions. It is particularly common among elderly medical and surgical patients and hospitalized and nursing home residents. Drugs with anticholinergic properties (e.g., diphenhydramine, which is present in some over-the-counter medications) and benzodiazepines may precipitate acute agitation and delirium in the elderly. Patients with dementia or other brain damage have a lower threshold for developing delirium and do so with greater frequency. Hallucinations are typically visual and accompanied by illusions (visual misinterpretation of things seen in the environment). Paranoid delusions may be present. The latter may be found in up to 40% of elderly patients with delirium. Physicians should suspect delirium in any elderly patient with an acute change in mental status, personality, or behavior. Delirium characterized by delusions, disordered thinking, and agitation must be distinguished from schizophrenia, schizophreniform disorder, or mania. The symptoms of mania overlap with those of delirium and sometimes occur secondary to a general medical condition. In delirium, the symptoms generally have an acute onset and tend to fluctuate over the course of the day; delusions are fragmented and unsystematized compared with schizophrenia or mania. In delirium, orientation or memory are usually impaired, in contrast to the other disorders. Treatment involves identification and treatment of the cause of delirium. Haloperidol may be useful for managing severe agitation and psychotic symptoms associated with delirium. Case reports of patients with delirium treated with risperidone, olanzapine, and quetiapine have indicated potential benefits. Prognosis of patients with psychotic symptoms associated with delirium is dependent largely on how quickly the underlying medical condition is identified and appropriately treated.

Psychoses Due to Medical Illnesses

DSM-IV criteria for a psychotic disorder caused by a general medical condition require prominent hallucinations or delusions, with evidence from the history, physical examination, or laboratory findings that the disturbance is the direct physiologic consequence of a general medical condition (Table 3–2). By definition,

Table 3–2. Medical and surgical causes of psychotic symptoms in the elderly

Neurologic	Parkinson's disease, epilepsy, subdural hematoma, stroke. Rarely: Huntington's disease, brain tumor
Infectious	Meningitis, encephalitis (e.g., herpes), syphilis, HIV/AIDS
Metabolic	B_{12} or folate deficiency, electrolyte imbalance (hyponatremia, hypocalcemia)
Endocrine	Thyroid disease, adrenal disease, hypo- or hyperglycemia

the disturbance is not better accounted for by another mental disorder and does not occur exclusively during the course of a delirium. Whether the predominant symptoms are delusions or hallucinations also is specified . Elders are at increased risk for such syndromes because of their higher rates of physical illnesses and resultant polypharmacy as well as their aging-related susceptibility to disruption of brain function (Marsh 1997). Usually, routine history and physical examination may suffice, but some cases are identified only by laboratory tests because psychotic symptoms may be the only overt manifestation. Physical illness has been reported to be very common at the onset of catatonic psychoses (Wilcox and Nasrallah 1986). The delusions may be related to specific neurological deficits such as anosagnosia, denial of blindness (Anton's syndrome), or reduplicative paramnesia (in which a patient claims to be present simultaneously in two locations). Aging patients with AIDS may develop central nervous system manifestations that often result in psychosis. The clinician must also consider acute viral encephalitis as a potential etiology of unexplained psychosis. If encephalitis is suspected, lumbar puncture should be performed after neuroimaging and electroencephalogram. Careful consideration of these varied etiologies is important for early diagnosis. Treatment involves identifying and correcting the underlying medical condition. Atypical antipsychotics may be necessary in some cases.

When psychosis develops in the context of epilepsy, the generally accepted first step is to maximize anticonvulsant therapy in an effort to reduce the possible contribution of electrophysiologic disturbances in the described areas (Arciniegas et al. 2001). When interictal psychosis persists despite such adjustments, initiation with low-dose atypical antipsychotics with the least potential for lowering the seizure threshold should be considered. Clozapine should be avoided due to its potential for seizures, especially at higher doses.

Psychoses Related to Parkinson's Disease

The incidence of psychotic symptoms in patients with Parkinson's disease (PD) ranges from 10% to 40%. The visual hallucinations and delusions appear to be multifactorial in origin and not entirely related to treatment (Barnes and David 2001; Holroyd et al. 2001). Higher doses of dopaminergic drugs (especially levodopa), disease severity, lower cognitive score, higher depression score, and worse visual acuity are important determinants of psychotic symptoms in patients with PD. Drug-induced psychosis increases in frequency as the disease progresses, particularly in patients with dementia. Chronic delusional psychosis with hallucinations occurring in patients with early onset PD may be the expression of a coexisting psychiatric illness that, prior to onset of the neurologic disease, had not been correctly diagnosed and has been disclosed by dopaminergic therapy (Cannas et al. 2001). Psychosis induced by dopamimetic agents appears to be dose related. Withdrawal of these agents is seldom considered because of the predictable aggravation of parkinsonian symptoms. Psychotic symptoms can be more disabling than the motor features of PD and can cause considerable caregiver distress. These symptoms pose a serious threat to the patient's ability to maintain independence.

Drug-induced psychoses consist of several distinct psychiatric syndromes that can be divided broadly into those occurring against a background of a clear sensorium and those accompanied by confusion and clouding of consciousness. Benign organic hallucinosis is the most common of these syndromes (30%). It usually occurs against a background of a clear sensorium and may not be a particularly troublesome problem if the patient is able to retain insight into the nature of these symptoms. More disabling syndromes usually include delusional thinking that is frequently paranoid, confusion, and even frank delirium. Although all of these psychotic syndromes can occur in isolation, mild symptoms tend to progress to more disabling ones if adequate and timely treatment is not instituted. Abnormal dreaming and sleep disruption often precede these difficulties by weeks to months and may provide an important early clue to their onset. Hallucinations in PD patients receiving chronic dopaminergic therapy can be persistent and progressive (Goetz et al. 2001). If reducing the dose of antiparkinsonian drugs is not feasible, low-dose antipsychotics with least potential for drug-induced parkinsonism should be considered. Low-dose clozapine remains the antipsychotic drug with a safety and efficacy profile best supported by scientific evidence (Poewe and Seppi 2001). In addition to its effects on psychosis, clozapine has been useful in reducing tremors and levodopa-induced dyskinesias in patients with PD. Clozapine has been effective at doses below 50 mg/day in 80%–90% of patients, with minimal effects on motor function. Open studies of risperidone in the treatment of psychosis in patients with PD have shown that 77% improved, but 28% developed significant motor worsening (Friedman and Factor 2000). Olanzapine in currently used doses of 2.5–15 mg/day seems to aggravate motor symptoms with lesser effect on psychosis compared with clozapine (Goetz et al. 2000; Poewe and Seppi 2001). In open studies of patients with PD, quetiapine resulted in improvement in psychosis in 85% of patients, and motor worsening was observed in only 13%, suggesting selective advantages of quetiapine in this population (Friedman and Factor 2000).

Psychotic Symptoms Associated With Ophthalmological Disorders

Visual hallucinations often accompany visual pathology or decreased visual acuity. Visual hallucinations have been described in association with various lesions at all levels of the visual system. Visual hallucinations due to ocular pathology are usually accompanied by decreased visual acuity and are not accompanied by delusions or auditory hallucinations; insight is typically retained. Visual hallucinations among patients with retinal disease are common, underdiagnosed, and not associated with cognitive deficits, abnormal personality traits, or a family or personal history of psychiatric morbidity (Scott et al. 2001). Correction of ocular pathology may resolve the hallucinations.

Psychosis Due to Prescription Drugs

When medication-induced psychosis occurs in the elderly, the most common offenders are antiparkinsonian drugs (levodopa, bromocriptine, amantadine); anticholinergic drugs (e.g., diphenhydramine); cimetidine, digoxin; antiarrhythmic drugs (lidocaine, quinidine, procainamide); and corticosteroids (Hubbard et al. 1991) (Table 3–3). Patients with dementia are very sensitive to medications with direct or indirect anticholinergic properties. Tactile hallucinations occur most commonly in toxic and metabolic disturbances or drug withdrawal states. Correct identification and removal of offending agents are usually sufficient to resolve psychotic symptoms due to drug toxicity. In some cases, atypical antipsychotics for a short period may be necessary.

Psychoses Related to Substance Abuse

Abuse and misuse of alcohol and psychoactive medications is common and adversely affects a growing proportion of the elderly population. Psychotic symptoms typically occur during acute intoxication and withdrawal. Elderly patients may not report alcohol or substance abuse to their clinicians. A high degree of suspicion, a thorough history (obtaining information from alternate sources such as a family member, home health worker, neighbor), use of screening questionnaires, and urine drug screens will identify most cases of psychoses due to drug or alcohol use disorder.

Psychoses Related to Alcohol Abuse

Psychotic symptoms can occur during alcohol withdrawal or intoxication and as a separate syndrome of alcohol-induced psychotic disorder with delusions (e.g., of infidelity) and/or hallucinations. Patients with alcoholic hallucinosis may resemble those with paranoid schizophrenia. Many patients with alcohol

---

Table 3–3. Medication and substance-induced psychotic symptoms in the elderly

Prescription medications
Antiparkinsonian drugs
    L-dopa or carbidopa
    Amantadine
    Bromocriptine
Anticholinergic and
  antihistaiminic agents
    Diphenhydramine
    Hydroxizine
Tricyclic antidepressants
Cimetidine
Stimulants
    Methylphenidate
    Amphetamine
    Thyroid
    Ephedrine
Analgesics and anti-
  inflammatory drugs
    Indomethacin
Antineoplastic agents
Oral or parenteral steroids
    Prednisone
    Dexamethasone
Antiarrythmic and cardiac drugs
    Digitalis
    Quinidine
    Procainamide
    Propranolol
Sedative-hypnotics
    Benzodiazepines
    Barbiturates
    Chloral hydrate

Over-the-counter medications
Antihistaminics
Cold medications
Cough suppressants
Sleep aids
Allergy medications

Substances of abuse
Alcohol
Cocaine
Opioids
Benzodiazepines
Cannabis

use disorder may have another psychiatric disorder (dual diagnoses). In older alcoholic persons, the coexisting problem is most commonly an affective or organic mental disorder, although anxiety disorders and schizophrenia also commonly coexist with alcoholism in older patients treated in general psychiatric clinic settings. Psychotic symptoms during withdrawal are treated using benzodiazepines and generally do not require antipsychotics. Identification and treatment of underlying comorbid medical and psychiatric condition may decrease risk of relapse.

Psychoses Related to Benzodiazepine Abuse

Benzodiazepines are disproportionately prescribed to older adults. Psychotic symptoms typically occur during abrupt withdrawal and are usually in the form of visual hallucinations and illusions. Treatment generally entails reinstitution of benzodiazepines with a more gradual taper.

Antipsychotics and Aging

The incidence of agranulocytosis and delirium associated with clozapine therapy appears to increase with age (Table 3–4). The cardiovascular side effects of clozapine (orthostatic hypotension, tachycardia, and rarely myocarditis) also limit its use in older patients. There is also a problem with sedation, risk of seizures, and anticholinergic toxicity. Risperidone may be associated with dose-dependent EPS, orthostasis, and peripheral edema. The most frequent treatment-emergent adverse events with olanzapine were somnolence, unsteady gait, and falls. Quetiapine is associated with risk of sedation and orthostasis, especially at higher doses. Problematic issues with use of ziprasidone in the elderly may be QTc prolongation and limited data on use.

Both conventional and atypical antipsychotics are associated with weight gain. Among the atypical agents, clozapine and olanzapine appear to have the greatest potential. Less weight is gained with the use of olanzapine in older compared with younger patients (Witterling and Mussigbrodt 1999). In a recent study, risperidone treatment for 1 year was not associated with weight gain among elderly persons with schizophrenia (Barak 2002). Atypical antipsychotics may be associated with new-onset diabetes, with risperidone having the lowest risk compared with clozapine, olanzapine, and quetiapine in patients age 40 and older (Sernyak et al. 2002).

Table 3–4. Antipsychotic dosing in the elderly

Antipsychotic medication	Dementia, dosage range per day (optimal dosage)	Schizophrenia and related disorders, dosage range per day (optimal dosage)
Risperidone	0.5–1.5 mg (1 mg)	1–3 mg (2 mg)
Olanzapine	5–10 mg (5 mg)	5–15 mg (higher in smokers) (10 mg)
Quetiapine	25–150 mg (?100 mg)	25–400 mg (?200 mg)
Ziprasidone	No data	No data in the elderly
Clozapine	6.25–50 mg (?25 mg)	50–300 mg (?100 mg)

Older patients usually require lower doses of medications, because aging is associated with reductions in renal clearance and volume of distribution. Concomitant medications, genetic variance in drug metabolism, and comorbid medical conditions may also alter the metabolism or excretion of psychotropic medications. Older patients may also be more sensitive to side effects because of greater end-organ sensitivity. All these factors should be considered in the risks and benefits assessment of psychotropics and in selecting an agent.

Risk of Tardive Dyskinesia

Older adults (especially with dementia) have a very high incidence of TDs (29% over 1 year to more than 60% over 3 years) with conventional antipsychotics (Jeste et al. 1995b, 1999). Risk of TDs with atypical antipsychotics is significantly lower (Beasley et al. 1999; Jeste et al. 2000). Early development of EPS is a strong predictor for TD in the elderly.

Polypharmacy

Whenever patients are taking more than one medication, the possibility of adverse drug–drug interactions should always be considered. Patients should be educated about the importance of informing their psychiatrist and other physicians about their current medications (including herbal remedies, non-herbal supplements and other over-the-counter drugs) whenever new medications are prescribed.

Conclusion

Psychotic symptoms in the elderly are highly prevalent, cause substantial morbidity and mortality, and can lead to premature institutionalization. They are eminently treatable. They incur enormous economic burden on society, especially if not diagnosed early and treated appropriately. In many cases, early treatment may prevent hospitalization and premature institutionalization. The etiology of late-life psychosis varies widely, making an accurate assessment of the problem and a determination of possible solutions somewhat difficult. Elderly patients with psychosis present treatment challenges. Psychosocial interventions are beneficial in all patients with psychotic disorders. Conventional antipsychotics have only a modest efficacy for psychosis in late life and frequent intolerable adverse effects, making them inadequate. Although the data on atypical antipsychotics in the elderly are not robust, sufficient data exist to indicate better efficacy and significantly reduced toxicity for these agents when used in appropriate doses. Although better than conventional antipsychotics, atypical antipsychotics are associated with significant adverse events and should be used judiciously. The limited literature available in several areas points to the need for further studies of late life psychotic disorders.

References

Alexopoulous GS, Silver JM, Kahn DA, et al: The Expert Consensus Guideline Series: agitation in older persons with dementia. Postgrad Med (special report):1–88, 1998

American Psychiatric Association: Diagnostic and Statistical Manual of Mental Disorders, 4th Edition Text Revision. Washington, DC, American Psychiatric Association, 2000

Arciniegas DB, Topkoff JL, Held K, et al: Psychosis due to neurologic conditions. Curr Treat Options Neurol 3:347–366, 2001

Ballard C, O'Brien J, Gray A, et al: Attention in patients with dementia with Lewy bodies and Alzheimer's disease. Arch Neurol 58:977–982, 2001

Barak Y: No weight gain among elderly schizophrenia patients after 1 year of risperidone treatment. J Clin Psychiatry 63:117–119, 2002

Barnes J, David AS: Visual hallucinations in Parkinson's disease: a review and phenomenological survey. J Neurol Neurosurg Psychiatry 70:727–733, 2001

Beasley CM, Dellva MA, Tamura RN, et al: Randomised double-blind comparison of the incidence of tardive dyskinesia in patients with schizophrenia during long-term treatment with olanzapine or haloperidol. Br J Psychiatry 174:23–30, 1999

Belitsky R, McGlashan TH: The manifestations of schizophrenia in late life: a dearth of data. Schizophr Bull 19:683–685, 1993

Brookmeyer R, Gray S: Methods for projecting the incidence and prevalence of chronic diseases in aging populations: application to Alzheimer's disease. Stat Med 19:1481–1493, 2000

Cannas A, Spissu A, Floris GL, et al: Chronic delusional hallucinatory psychosis in early onset Parkinson's disease: drug-induced complication or sign of an idiopathic psychiatric illness? Neurol Sci 22:53–54, 2001

Christenson R, Blazer D: Epidemiology of persecutory ideation in an elderly population in the community. Am J Psychiatry 141:1088–1091, 1984

Ciompi L: The natural history of schizophrenia in the long term. Br J Psychiatry 136:277–286, 1980

Cummings JL: ChEIs: a new class of psychotropic compounds. Am J Psychiatry 157:4–15, 2000

Cummings JC, Miller B, Hill MA: Neuropsychiatric aspects of multi-infarct dementia and dementia of the Alzheimer's type. Arch Neurology 44:389–393, 1987

DeDyn PP, Rabheru K, Rasmussen A, et al: A randomized trial of risperidone, placebo, and haloperidol for behavioral symptoms of dementia. Neurology 53:946–955, 1999

Farber NB, Rubin EH, Newcomer JW, et al: Increased neocortical neurofibrillary tangle density in subjects with Alzheimer disease and psychosis. Arch Gen Psychiatry 57:1165–1173, 2000

Feinstein A, Ron MA: Psychosis associated with demonstrable brain disease. Psychol Med 20:793–803, 1990

Flint AJ, Rifat SL: Two-year outcome of psychotic depression in late life. Am J Psychiatry 155:178–183, 1998

Friedman JH, Factor SA: Atypical antipsychotics in the treatment of drug-induced psychosis in Parkinson's disease. Mov Disord 15:201–211, 2000

Gilmore J, McGuire G, Kennedy JS, et al: Acute double-blind comparison of olanzapine and haloperidol in schizophrenia patients age 60 and older. Poster abstract 71, presented at the annual meeting of the American Association of Geriatric Psychiatry, Orlando, FL, February 2002

Goetz CG, Blasucci LM, Leurgans S, et al: Olanzapine and clozapine: comparative effects on motor function in hallucinating Parkinson's disease patients. Neurology 55:789–794, 2000

Goetz CG, Leurgans S, Pappert EJ, et al: Prospective longitudinal assessment of hallucinations in Parkinson's disease. Neurology 57:2078–2082, 2001

Goldberg RJ: Long-term use of risperidone for the treatment of dementia-related behavioral disturbances in a nursing home population. Int J Geriatr Psychopharmacol 2:1–4, 1999

Grossberg GT, Manepalli J: The older patient with psychotic symptoms. Psychiatr Serv 46:55–59, 1995

Gurland BJ, Cross PS: Epidemiology of psychopathology in old age. Psychiatr Clin North Am 5:11–26, 1982

Harvey PD, Silverman JM, Mohs RC, et al: Cognitive decline in late-life schizophrenia: a longitudinal study of geriatric chronically hospitalized patients. Biol Psychiatry 45:32–40, 1999

Harvey PD, Mao L, Napolitano J, et al: Improved cognition in elderly schizophrenic patients: risperidone versus olanzapine. Ma4. Presented at annual meeting of American Association of Geriatric Psychiatry, Orlando, FL, February 2002

Heaton RK, Gladsjo JA, Palmer BW, et al: Stability and course of neuropsychological deficits in schizophrenia. Arch Gen Psychiatry 58:24–32, 2001

Henderson AS, Kay DWK: The epidemiology of functional psychoses of late onset. Eur Arch Psychiat Clinn Neurosci 247:176–189, 1997

Henderson AS, Korten AE, Levings C, et al: Psychotic symptoms in the elderly: a prospective study in a population sample. Int J Geriatr Psychiatry 13:484–492, 1998

Hirono N, Mori E, Tanimukai S, et al: Distinctive neurobehavioral features among neurodegenerative dementias. J Neuropsychiatry Clin Neurosci 11:498–503, 1999

Holroyd S, Shepherd ML, Hunter Downs J III: Occipital atrophy is associated with visual hallucinations in Alzheimer's disease. J Neuropsychiatry Clin Neurosci 12:25–28, 2000

Holroyd S, Currie L, Wooten GF. Prospective study of hallucinations and delusions in Parkinson's disease. J Neurol Neurosurg Psychiatry 70:734–738, 2001

Howanitz E, Pardo M, Smelson DA, et al: The efficacy and safety of clozapine versus chlorpromazine in geriatric schizophrenia. J Clin Psychiatry 60:41–44, 1999

Howard R, Rabins PV, Seeman MV, et al: Late-onset schizophrenia and very-late-onset schizophrenia-like psychosis: an international consensus. The International Late-Onset Schizophrenia Group. Am J Psychiatry 157:172–178, 2000

Hubbard JR, Levenson JL, Patrick GA: Psychiatric side effects associated with the ten most commonly dispensed prescription drugs: a review. J Fam Pract 33:177–186, 1991

Jeste DV, Lacro JP, Gilbert PL, et al: Treatment of late-life schizophrenia with neuroleptics. Schizophr Bull 19:817–830, 1993

Jeste DV, Gilbert PL, McAdams LA, et al: Considering neuroleptic maintenance and taper on a continuum: need for individual rather than dogmatic approach. Arch Gen Psychiatry 52:209–212, 1995a

Jeste DV, Caligiuri MP, Paulsen JS, et al: Risk of tardive dyskinesia in older patients: a prospective longitudinal study of 266 outpatients. Arch Gen Psychiatry 52:756–765, 1995b

Jeste DV, Symonds LL, Harris JM, et al: Nondementia nonpraecox dementia praecox? Am J Geriatr Psychiatry 5:302–317, 1997

Jeste DV, Rockwell E, Harris MJ, et al: Conventional vs. newer antipsychotics in elderly patients. Am J Geriatr Psychiatry 7:70–76, 1999

Jeste DV, Okamoto A, Napolitano J, et al: Low incidence of persistent tardive dyskinesia in elderly patients with dementia treated with risperidone. Am J Psychiatry 157:1150–1155, 2000

Katz IR, Jeste DV, Mintzer JE, et al: Comparison of risperidone and placebo for psychosis and behavioral disturbances associated with dementia: a randomized, double-blind trial. J Clin Psychiatry 60:107–115, 1999

Leuchter AF, Spar JE: The late-onset psychoses: clinical and diagnostic features. J Nerv Ment Dis 173:488–494, 1985

Madhusoodanan S, Brecher M, Brenner R, et al: Risperidone in the treatment of elderly patients with psychotic disorders. Am J Geriatr Psychiatry 7:132–138, 1999

Marsh CM: Psychiatric presentations of medical illness. Psychiatr Clin North Am 20:181–204, 1997

McKeith I, Del Ser T, Anand R, et al: Rivastigmine provides symptomatic benefit in dementia with Lewy bodies: findings from a placebo-controlled international multicenter study. Lancet 356:2031–2036, 2000

Mega MS, Lee L, Dinov ID, et al: Cerebral correlates of psychotic symptoms in Alzheimer's disease. J Neurol Neurosurg Psychiatry 69:167–171, 2000

Meyers BS: Geriatric delusional depression. Clin Geratr Med 8:299–308, 1992

Meyers BS: Treatment of psychotic depression, in Geriatric Psychopharmacology, 9th Edition. Edited by Nelson JC. New York, Marcel Dekker, 1998, pp 99–114

Meyers BS, Klimstra SA, Gabriele M, et al: Continuation treatment of delusional depression in older adults. Am J Geriatr Psychiatry 9:415–422, 2001

McManus DQ, Arvanitis LA, Kowalcyk BB: Quetiapine, a novel antipsychotic: experience in elderly patients with psychotic disorders. J Clin Psychiatry 60:292–298, 1999

Neuropathology Group of the Medical Research Council Cognitive Function and Ageing Study (MRC CFAS): Papthological correlates of late-onset dementia in a multicentre, community-based population in England and Wales. Lancet 357:169–175, 2001

Ostling S, Skoog I: Psychotic symptoms and paranoid ideation in a non-demented population-based sample of the very old. Arch Gen Psychiatry 59:53–59, 2002

Palmer BW, Heaton SC, Jeste DV: Older patients with schizophrenia: challenges in the coming decades. Psychiatr Serv 50:1178–1183, 1999

Palmer BW, McClure FS, Jeste DV: Schizophrenia in late life: findings challenge traditional concepts. Harv Rev Psychiatry 9:51–58, 2001

Paulsen JS, Salmon DP, Thal LJ, et al: Incidence of and risk factors for hallucinations and delusions in patients with probable AD. Neurology 54:1965–1971, 2000

Poewe W, Seppi K: Treatment Options for Depression and Psychosis in Parkinson's Disease. J Neurol 248(suppl 3):12–21, 2001

Pollock BG, Mulsant BH, Rosen J, et al: Comparison of citalopram, perphenazine, and placebo for the acute treatment of psychosis and behavioral disturbances in hospitalized, demented patients. Am J Psychiatry 159:460–465, 2002

Sajatovic M, Ramirez LF, Garver D, et al: Clozapine therapy for older veterans. Psychiatr Serv 49:340–344, 1998

Schneider LS, Pollock VE, Lyness S: A meta-analysis of controlled trials of neuroleptic treatments in dementia. J Am Geriatr Soc 38:553–563, 1990

Scott IU, Schein OD, Feuer W, et al: Visual hallucinations in patients with retinal disease. Am J Ophthalmol 131:590–598, 2001

Sernyak MJ, Leslie DL, Alarcon RD, et al: Association of diabetes mellitus with use of atypical neuroleptics in the treatment of schizophrenia. Am J Psychiatry 159:561–566, 2002

Soares JC, Gershon S: Therapeutic targets in late-life psychoses: review of concepts and critical issues. Schizophr Res 27:227–239, 1997

Speer DC, Bates K: Comorbid mental and substance disorders among older psychiatric patients. J Am Geriatr Soc 40:886–890, 1992

Street JS, Tollefson GD, Tohen M, et al: Olanzapine for psychotic conditions in the elderly. Psychiatr Ann 30:191–196, 2000a

Street J, Clark WS, Gannonks KS, et al: Olanzapine treatment of psychotic and behavioral symptoms in patients with Alzheimer's disease in nursing care facilities. Arch Gen Psychiatry 57:968–976, 2000b

Sultzer DL: Neuroimaging and the origin of psychiatric symptoms in dementia. Int Psychogeriatr 8(suppl 3):239–243, 1996

Sweet RA, Nimgaonkar VL, Kamboh MI, et al: Dopamine receptor genetic variation, psychosis, and aggression in Alzheimer's disease. Arch Neurol 55:1335–1340, 1998

Sweet RA, Hamilton RL, Healy MT, et al: Alteration of striatal dopamine receptor binding in Alzheimer disease are associated with Lewy body pathology and antemortem psychosis. Arch Neurol 58:466–472, 2001

Sweet RA, Nimgaonkar VL, Devlin B, et al: Increased familial risk of the psychotic phenotype of Alzheimer disease. Neurology 58:907–911, 2002

Targum SD, Abbott JL: Psychoses in the elderly: a spectrum of disorders. J Clin Psychiatry 60(suppl 8):4–10, 1990

Tariot PN, Salzman C, Yeung PP, et al: Long-term use of quetiapine in elderly patients with psychotic disorders. Clin Ther 22:1068–1084, 2000

Thorpe L: The treatment of psychotic disorders in late life. Can J Psychiatry 1:19S–27S, 1997

Umapathy C, Mulsant BH, Pollock BG: Bipolar disorder in the elderly. Psychiatr Ann 30:473–480, 2000

Van Gerpen MW, Johnson JE, Winstead DK: Mania in the geriatric patient population: a review of the literature. Am J Geriatr Psychiatry 7:188–202, 1999

Verma S, Orengo CA, Kunik ME, et al: Tolerability and effectiveness of atypical antipsychotics in male geriatric inpatients. Int J Geriatr Psychiatry 16:223–227, 2001

Webster J, Grossberg GT: Late-life onset of psychotic symptoms. Am J Geriatr Psychiatry 6:196–202, 1998

Wilcox JA, Nasrallah HA: Organic factors in catatonia. Br J Psychiatry 149:782–784, 1986

Witterling T, Mussigbrodt HE: Weight gain: side effect of atypical neuroleptics. J Clin Psychopharmacol 19:316–321, 1999

Chapter 4

Late-Life Addictions

Frederic C. Blow, Ph.D.
David W. Oslin, M.D.

Introduction

There is growing interest in targeted disease prevention and in efforts to promote healthy lifestyles across all age groups as a means to reduce disability and health care costs. Because of the increased incidence of health care problems, the growing population of older adults is more likely to seek health care on a regular or semi-regular basis than are younger adults. This fact is responsible for high health care costs among the elderly (Barry 1997; Fuchs 1999; Krop et al. 1998; Schneider and Guralnik 1990; Waldo et al. 1989). Many of the acute and chronic medical and psychiatric conditions experienced by older adults are influenced by their lifestyle choices and behaviors, such as the consumption of alcohol. Excessive alcohol use is associated with several adverse health effects in this population, including greater risk for harmful drug interactions, injury, depression, memory problems, liver disease, cardiovascular disease, cognitive changes, and sleep problems (Barry 1997; Gambert and Katsoyannis 1995; Liberto et al. 1992; Wetle 1997).

It has recently been suggested that a focus on lifestyle factors, including the use of alcohol, may be the most appropriate way to maximize health outcomes and minimize health care costs among older adults (Barry et al. 2001; Blow 1998; Wetle 1997). Thus, systematic alcohol screening and intervention methods are particularly relevant to providing high-quality health care to older adults, especially in settings such as mental health clinics, rehabilitation clinics, and emergency departments. Older adults with alcohol-related problems are a special and vulnerable population who require elder-specific screening and intervention procedures focused on the unique issues associated with drinking in later life. Problems related to alcohol use are by far the largest class of substance use problems seen in older adults today. In addition, as the baby-boom generation ages, providers may begin to see a greater number of patients who use illicit drugs than has been seen in previous cohorts. As a result, there will be an increasing need to develop screening and interventions for older adults with illicit drug problems.

In the coming decades, the aging of the baby-boom generation is likely to have an enormous impact on the need and demand for health care among older adults (Day 1996). Despite significant advances made in the past two decades both in the understanding of the aging process, with its attendant health problems, and in the understanding and consequences of alcohol problems and alcoholism, little attention has been paid to the intersection of the fields of gerontology or geriatrics and alcohol studies. In recent years, however, there has been an increased interest in alcohol and other substance abuse problems among the elderly and its effects on this now-aging population. This chapter reviews the latest research on the identification, effects, and treatment of late-life addictions.

Prevalence of the Problem

Prevalence estimates of problem drinking among older adults, based on community survey results, have ranged from 1% to 15% (Adams et al. 1996; Gurland and Cross 1982; Robins et al. 1984; Schuckit and Pastor 1978). These rates vary widely depending on the definition of risk drinking or alcohol abuse/dependence and on the methodology used in obtaining samples. Overall, among clinical populations, estimates of alcohol abuse/dependence are substantially higher because problem drinkers of all ages are more likely to present in health care settings (Institute of Medicine 1990).

Most older adults who drink at high-risk levels have not been recognized as at-risk or problem drinkers by health care personnel (Adams et al. 1996; Blow et al. 2000). Additionally, very few older patients with alcohol abuse or dependence seek help in specialized addiction treatment settings. However, because older adults generally seek medical care on a more regular basis than younger adults, health care providers in general medical settings are crucial in identifying those older adults in their care who may need assistance with at-risk or problem drinking. Older adults may also be more likely to seek help in a mental health setting for alcohol-related symptoms such as depression rather than seek care in an addiction clinic (Oslin et al. 1999).

The rates of illegal drug abuse in the current elderly cohort are very low (Blow 1998). However, misuse and inappropriate use of prescription medications is a substantial issue in this population, with multiple determinants, causes, and consequences. Most misuse can be treated outside of specialized substance abuse treatment programs through education of patients, families, and providers. Psychoactive drug misuse and abuse is one exception and may require additional specialized treatment.

Drinking Guidelines

Older adults have an increased sensitivity to alcohol as well as to over-the-counter and prescription medications compared with younger adults (Adams 1995). There is an age-related decrease in lean body mass versus total volume of fat, and the resultant decrease in total body volume increases the total distribution of alcohol and other mood-altering chemicals in the body. The liver enzymes that metabolize alcohol and certain other drugs are less efficient with age, and central nervous system sensitivity increases with age (Adams 1995). Of particular concern in this age group is the potential interaction of medication and alcohol. For some patients, any alcohol use coupled with the use of specific over-the-counter or prescription medications can be problematic.

Because of these factors, alcohol use recommendations for older adults are generally lower than those set for adults under age 65. The National Institute on Alcohol Abuse and Alcoholism (NIAAA) and the Center for Substance Abuse Treatment's (CSAT) Treatment Improvement Protocol (TIP) for older adults (Blow 1998; Dufour and Fuller 1995; National Institute on Alcohol Abuse and Alcoholism 1995) recommend that persons age 65 and older consume

- No more than one standard drink per day or seven standard drinks per week.
- No more than two standard drinks on any drinking day.
- Less than 1 standard drink per day for women.

A *standard drink* is defined as one 12-oz bottle of beer, one 4-oz glass of wine, 1.5 oz (a shot) of liquor (e.g., vodka, gin, whiskey), or 4 oz of liqueur. These recommendations have been shown to be consistent with data regarding the relationship between consumption of alcohol and alcohol-related problems in this age group (Chermack et al. 1996). Drinking that exceeds these limits increases the risk of alcohol-related problems, including DSM-IV-TR symptoms (American Psychiatric Association 2000; Chermack et al. 1996). They are also consistent with the current evidence on the beneficial health effects of drinking (Doll et al. 1994; Klatsky et al. 1997; Poikolainen 1991). The cardioprotective and possibly cerebrovascular-protective effects of alcohol have been associated with consumption of 1–2 standard drinks per day. However, the research and clinical controversy regarding the risks versus the benefits of moderate alcohol use for elderly populations continues.

Screening and Assessment

The expert panel for the TIP series #26, *Substance Abuse Among Older Adults* (Blow 1998), recommended that every person age 65 and older be screened for alcohol and prescription drug use/abuse as part of regular medical and psychiatric care and that patients should be screened again yearly if certain physical or emotional symptoms emerge (see "Medical and Psychiatric Comorbidities" later in this chapter) or if the person is undergoing major life changes or transitions.

The goals of screening are 1) to identify at-risk drinkers, problem drinkers, or persons with alcohol dependence; and 2) to determine whether further assessment is necessary. The rationale for such screening is the high incidence of alcohol use and abuse problems in this population, which justifies the cost, as well as the fact that alcohol can adversely affect morbidity and mortality and that effective treatments and valid, cost-effective methods for screening are available.

Assessment of substance use, misuse, and abuse should be part of a thorough history, physical, and laboratory examination. Clinicians can obtain accurate histories by asking questions about the recent past, embedding alcohol-use questions in the context of other health behaviors (e.g., exercise, weight, smoking), and paying attention to nonverbal cues that the patient is minimizing use. Common signs and symptoms of substance misuse in older adults are listed in Table 4–1. Alcohol screening questions can be asked by verbal interview, by paper-and-pencil questionnaire, or by computerized questionnaire; all three methods are reliable and valid (Barry and Fleming 1990; Greist et al. 1987). It is sometimes easier and more effective to ask initial screening questions in questionnaire format and to save follow-up questions for the actual interview with the patient. Any positive responses can lead to further questions about consequences. To successfully incorporate alcohol and drug screening into health care practices, such screening should be simple and should be consistent with other screening procedures already in place (Barry and Blow 1999). In addition to quantifying the frequency and quantity of use, instruments such as the Short Michigan Alcohol Screening Test-Geriatric version (SMAST-G; Blow et al. 1992), the Alcohol Use Disorders Test (AUDIT), or the Alcohol Related Problems Survey (ARPS; Moore et al. 2000).

Screening for alcohol use and problems is not always standardized, and not all standardized instruments have good reliability and validity in older adults. For example, the CAGE, a widely used alcohol screening test, does not have high validity with older adults (Adams et al. 1996) and, if used, should be part of a larger questionnaire or interview that includes quantity and frequency questions as well as questions about consequences. The SMAST-G (Table 4–2) and quantity/frequency questions (Table 4–3) have the greatest validity and reliability in this population. A combination of these two instruments provides the best overall picture of a potential problem. The SMAST-G was developed specifically for older adults and is useful both as a screening

Table 4–1. Signs and symptoms of potential alcohol problems in older adults

Anxiety	Increased tolerance to alcohol
Blackouts, dizziness	Legal difficulties
Depression	Memory loss
Disorientation	New difficulties in decision making
Excessive mood swings	Poor hygiene
Falls, bruises, burns	Poor nutrition
Family problems	Seizures, idiopathic
Financial problems	Sleep problems
Headaches	Social isolation
Incontinence	Unusual response to medications

Source. Adapted from Fleming and Barry 1992 and Barry et al. 2001

tool and to track progress in treatment. Included in the initial assessment is the patient's potential to experience acute withdrawal. Severe withdrawal, such as that from alcohol use, can be life threatening and warrants careful attention. Patients with severe symptoms of dependency or withdrawal and patients with significant medical or psychiatric comorbidity may require inpatient hospitalization for acute stabilization prior to implementing an outpatient management strategy.

Many prescription medications have serious and potentially life-threatening interactions with alcohol (Adams 1995; Blow 1998). Table 4–4 lists common medications with significant alcohol interactions. When assessing patients for alcohol problems, a careful review of all medications being taken should be conducted, especially for patients reporting any alcohol use. Specific advice about the dangers of combining alcohol with prescription and over-the-counter medications, especially psychoactive agents, should be given and regularly reinforced (Blow 1998).

Problems With DSM-IV-TR Criteria for Older Adults

Most behavioral health providers use the model defined in DSM-IV-TR for classifying the signs and symptoms of alcohol-related

Table 4–2. Short Michigan Alcoholism Screening Test—Geriatric version

	Yes (1)	No (0)
1. When talking with others, do you ever underestimate how much you actually drink?	___	___
2. After a few drinks, have you sometimes not eaten or been able to skip a meal because you didn't feel hungry?	___	___
3. Does having a few drinks help decrease your shakiness or tremors?	___	___
4. Does alcohol sometimes make it hard for you to remember parts of the day or night?	___	___
5. Do you usually take a drink to relax or calm your nerves?	___	___
6. Do you drink to take your mind off your problems?	___	___
7. Have you ever increased your drinking after experiencing a loss in your life?	___	___
8. Has a doctor or nurse ever said they were worried or concerned about your drinking?	___	___
9. Have you ever made rules to manage your drinking?	___	___
10. When you feel lonely, does having a drink help?	___	___
Total SMAST-G score (0–10)	___	

Scoring: Two or more "Yes" responses is indicative of an alcohol problem.

Note. For further information, contact Frederic C. Blow, Ph.D., at the University of Michigan Alcohol Research Center, 400 E. Eisenhower Parkway, Suite A., Ann Arbor, MI 48108, 734–761–2210.
Source. Copyright 1991, The Regents of the University of Michigan.

problems. DSM-IV-TR uses specific criteria to distinguish between those drinkers who abuse alcohol and those who are dependent on alcohol.

Although widely used, the DSM-IV-TR criteria may not apply to many older adults who experience neither the legal, social, nor

Table 4–3. Quantity/frequency questions

1. In the past 3 months, have you been drinking alcoholic drinks at all (e.g., beer, wine, wine cooler, sherry, gin, vodka or other hard liquor)? ____Yes ____No

If **Yes**,

In the past 3 months, on average, how many <u>days per week</u> have you been drinking alcohol?

None 1 2 3 4 5 6 7

On a day when you have had alcohol to drink, <u>how many drinks</u> have you had?

1 2 3 4 5 6 7 8 9 10 11 12 13 14 or more

2. In the past 3 months, how many times have you had four or more drinks on an occasion?

None 1 2 3 4 5 6 7 8 9 10 or more

Scoring based on quantity/frequency <u>and</u> binge drinking:

Quantity X frequency = score

Men and women age 65 and older:

    Eight or more drinks/week or

    Two or more occasions of binge drinking (four or more drinks/ occasion) in past month

---

psychological consequences specified. For example, "failure to fulfill major role obligations at work, school, or home" is less applicable to a retired person with minimal familial responsibilities; nor does the criterion "continued use of the substance(s) despite persistent or recurrent problems" always apply. Many older alcoholics do not realize that their persistent or recurrent problems are related to their drinking, a view likely to be reinforced by health care clinicians who attribute these problems, in whole or in part, to the aging process or to age-related comorbidities.

Although tolerance is one DSM-IV-TR criterion for a diagnosis of substance dependence, the thresholds of consumption often considered by clinicians as indicative of tolerance may be set too high for older adults because of their altered sensitivity to and body distribution of alcohol (Atkinson 1990). Intolerance to alcohol does not necessarily mean that an older adult does not have a drinking problem or is not experiencing serious negative effects

Table 4–4. Psychoactive medications with significant alcohol interactions

Drug	Brand name
Anxiolytics	
Benzodiazepines	
Alprazolam	Xanax
Chlordiazepoxide	Librium
Diazepam	Valium
Lorazepam	Ativan
Oxazepam	Serax
Clonazepam	Klonopin
Buspirone	BuSpar
Meprobamate	Miltown
Sedative/Hypnotics	
Benzodiazepines	
Flurazepam	Dalmane
Prazepam	Centrax
Quazepam	Doral
Temazepam	Restoril
Triazolam	Halcion
Other sedatives	
Zolpidem	Ambien
Chloral hydrate	Noctec
Hydroxyzine	Atarax
Diphenhydramine	Benadryl
Doxylamine	Unisom
Glutethimide	
Opiate/Opioid analgesics	
Methylmorphine	Morphine
Codeine	Tylenol III, Robitussin A-C
Hydrocodone	Lortab
Meperidine	Demerol
Oxycodone	Percodan/Percocet
Propoxyphene	Darvon
Pentazocine	Talwin

A number of brief alcohol intervention studies have been conducted in primary care settings with younger adults (e.g., Chick et al. 1985; Fleming et al. 1997; Kristenson et al. 1983; Persson and Magnusson 1989), with primarily positive results. Both brief interventions and brief therapies have been shown to be effective in a range of clinical settings (Barry 1999). These trials have employed various approaches to change drinking behaviors, ranging from relatively unstructured counseling and feedback to more formal structured interventions adults (Chick et al. 1985; Fleming et al. 1997; Kristenson et al. 1983; Persson and Magnusson 1989), and have relied heavily on concepts and techniques from the behavioral self-control training (BSCT) literature (Miller and Hester 1986; Miller and Munoz 1976; Miller and Rollnick 2002; Miller and Taylor 1980).

Drinking goals of the brief treatment intervention have been flexible, allowing the individual, with guidance from the provider, to choose drinking in moderation or abstinence. The goal of brief counseling is to motivate problem drinkers to change their behavior. Studies of brief interventions have avoided labeling individuals as alcoholic or as suffering from alcoholism. Babor et al. (1994) pointed out that the use of such terms may be inappropriate for at-risk drinkers.

To date, two brief alcohol intervention trials have been conducted with older adults. Fleming et al. (1999) and Blow et al. (Blow FC, Barry KL, Walton MA: "The Health Profile Project," unpublished, June 2000) have conducted randomized clinical brief intervention trials to reduce hazardous drinking in older adults using advice protocols in primary care settings. These studies have shown that older adults can be engaged in brief intervention protocols, that the protocols are acceptable in this population, and that drinking is reduced among the at-risk drinkers receiving the interventions compared with those in a control group.

The study by Fleming's group was a randomized, controlled clinical trial conducted in Wisconsin with 24 community-based primary care practices (43 practitioners) located in 10 counties. Of the patients screened for problem drinking, 105 men and 53 women met inclusion criteria ($n=158$) and were randomized into either a control ($n=71$) or an intervention group ($n=87$). The intervention consisted of two, 10–15 minute physician-delivered counseling visits that included advice, education, and contracting using a scripted workbook. No significant differences were found between the groups at baseline on alcohol use, age, socioeconomic status, smoking status, rates of depression or anxiety, frequency of conduct disorders, lifetime drug use, or health care utilization. At baseline, both groups consumed an average of 15 or 16 drinks per week. At 12-month follow-up, the intervention group drank significantly less than the control group ($P<0.001$).

The study by Blow and colleagues, which was a larger, elder-specific study, is currently being finalized in primary care settings located in southeast Michigan (Maixner et al. 1999). The intervention in use involves both brief advice discussion by either a psychologist or social worker, as used in the World Health Organization studies, and motivational interviewing techniques (Miller and Rollnick 2002), including feedback. A total of 452 subjects were randomized in this trial, with over 26% of African American race. The study found preliminary results similar to those of the Fleming et al. study in terms of 7-day alcohol use and binge drinking at 12-month follow-up.

These randomized controlled clinical trials extend the positive results of trials with younger at-risk drinkers to even more vulnerable populations of older adults.

Referral to Specialized Treatment

Some patients with more severe problems or who do not respond well to the recommendations given as part of brief interventions may need services found in more traditional specialty addiction programs. These services might include more formalized detoxification programs, group therapy, and case management or formalized psychotherapy. In addition, in patients with complex symptoms such as comorbid depression or anxiety, consultation from mental health specialists can be extremely useful.

There are two important considerations when referring patients to other providers. First, referrals are conducted either to assist in the management of the patient or as a consultation.

Thus, referrals are usually done when patients are not meeting their goals and the primary providers seek the opinion of specialists to help the patients meet these goals. When considering referral sources for elderly patients, providers will consider, among other things, the social, emotional, and financial resources of the patient and the referral site location. Older patients may have special circumstances such as transportation, mobility, or financial problems that limit where they can go for care. The best referral sources have some experience with older adults. Realistically, however, substance abuse specialists who have experience working with older adults are not available in every community. A supportive, empathetic approach provides the patient with the best opportunity for success.

Detoxification and Withdrawal

Alcohol withdrawal symptoms commonly occur in patients who stop drinking or markedly cut down their drinking after regular heavy use. Alcohol withdrawal can range from mild and almost unnoticeable symptoms to severe and life-threatening ones. The classical set of symptoms associated with alcohol withdrawal includes autonomic hyperactivity (increased pulse rate, increased blood pressure, increased temperature), restlessness, disturbed sleep, anxiety, nausea, and tremor. More severe withdrawal can be manifested by auditory, visual, or tactile hallucinations; delirium; seizures; and coma. Other substances of abuse such as benzodiazepines, opioids, and cocaine have distinct withdrawal symptoms that are also potentially life threatening. Elderly patients have been shown to have a longer duration of withdrawal symptoms and withdrawal has the potential for complicating other medical and psychiatric illnesses. No evidence exists, however, to suggest that older patients are more prone to alcohol withdrawal or need longer treatment for withdrawal symptoms (Brower et al. 1994).

Due to the potential for life-threatening complications, all clinicians caring for patients with substance abuse need to have a fundamental understanding of withdrawal symptoms and the potential complications. A standardized assessment of withdrawal such as the Revised Clinical Institute Withdrawal Assessment for Alcohol Scale (Foy et al. 1988; Sullivan et al. 1989), developed for use with patients of all ages, can be particularly useful for providers.

Specialized Substance Abuse Treatment

Very few systematic studies of formal alcoholism treatment outcome among older adults have been published (Atkinson 1995). The study of treatment outcomes for older adults who meet criteria for alcohol abuse or dependence has become a critical issue because of these patients' unique needs for targeted treatment intervention. Traditional residential alcoholism treatment programs generally provide services to few older adults; thus, sample size issues have been a barrier to studying treatment outcomes for older adults in specialized treatment programs. The development of elder-specific alcoholism treatment programs has provided more opportunity to study larger samples of this special population (Atkinson 1995). A final limitation when studying older adults in substance abuse treatment programs is the lack of longitudinal assessments of treatment outcome. More research is needed to determine whether elder-specific programs show better outcomes than mixed-age programs.

Traditionally, outpatient substance abuse treatment has been reserved for specialized clinics focused only on substance abuse. It is becoming increasingly apparent that this model is inadequate for addressing the broader public health demand. There is a need to involve a variety of clinicians and clinical settings in the delivery of substance abuse treatment, particularly in the case of older adults with concurrent depression who rarely seek specialized addiction services. The traditional addiction clinic focuses on supportive group psychotherapy and encourages patients to attend regular self-help group meetings such as Alcoholics Anonymous (AA), Alcoholics Victorious, Rational Recovery, or Narcotics Anonymous. For older adults, peer-specific group activities are considered superior to mixed-age group activities. Individual psychosocial support is also very effective in the treatment of late-life alcoholism (Oslin et al. 2002).

Outpatient rehabilitation, in addition to focusing on active addiction issues, usually needs to address issues of time management. Abstinence reduces the time spent maintaining the substance use disorder. The management of this time, which is often the greater part of a patient's day, is critical to the progress of treatment. Use of resources such as day programs and senior centers can be beneficial, especially in cognitively impaired patients. Social services such as financial support are often needed to stabilize the patient in early recovery. Supervised living arrangements such as halfway houses, group homes, nursing homes, and residence with relatives should also be considered.

The use of medications to support abstinence may be of benefit but is not well studied. No research to date has addressed pharmacological treatment of older alcoholics, although studies are under way using naltrexone as well as various antidepressants, including the selective serotonin reuptake inhibitors (SSRIs). Some of the general principles used in treating younger patients should be applied to older patients as well. For example, benzodiazepines are important in the treatment of alcohol detoxification but have no clinical relevance for maintaining long-term abstinence because of their abuse potential and the potential for fostering further alcohol or benzodiazepine abuse. Disulfiram may benefit some well-motivated patients, but cardiac and hepatic disease limits the use of this agent in the elderly (Blow 1998).

Treatment Compliance Studies

Most treatment outcome research on older adults with substance use disorders has focused on compliance with treatment program expectations, in particular the patient's fulfillment of prescribed treatment activities and goals, including drinking behavior (Atkinson 1995). Results from compliance studies have shown that age-specific programming improved treatment completion and resulted in higher rates of attendance at group meetings compared with mixed-age treatment (Atkinson et al. 1993). In addition, older adults with substance use disorders were significantly more likely to complete treatment than younger patients (Schuckit and Pastor 1978; Wiens et al. 1982). Atkinson et al. (1993) also found that the proportion of older men completing treatment was twice that of younger men.

Age of onset of alcohol problems has been a major focus of research for elderly treatment compliance studies in the elderly. In a study by Schonfeld and Dupree (1991) using a matched-pairs, post hoc design, rates of completion of 6-month day treatment for 23 older male and female alcoholics (age 55 and older) whose problem drinking began before age 50 (early onset) were compared with 23 alcoholics who began problem drinking after age 50 (late onset). Late-onset problem drinkers were significantly more likely to complete treatment, although in a subsequent report that included the larger sample of 148 from which these patients were selected, no difference was found in completion rate based on age of onset.

In another study of 132 male alcoholic veterans 60 years of age and older, the sample was divided into the following subgroups: early onset (age 40 and younger, $n=50$), midlife onset (age 41–59, $n=62$), and late onset (age 60 and older, $n=20$) (Atkinson et al. 1990). Age of onset was related to program completion and to weekly meeting attendance, with the late-onset subgroup showing the best compliance. However, a subsequent analysis of 128 men age 55 and older in alcoholism treatment found that drinking relapses during treatment were unrelated to age of onset (Atkinson et al. 1993). Furthermore, onset age did not contribute significantly to variance in program completion but was related to meeting attendance rate. Studies on the effect of age of onset on treatment compliance have yielded mixed results.

In a study of treatment matching, Rice et al. (1993) compared drinking outcomes for randomly assigned male and female alcoholics 3 months after beginning one of three age-mixed outpatient treatment protocols scheduled to last for 4 months. The sample included 42 individuals age 50 years and older, 134 patients age 30–49, and 53 patients age 18–29. There were no main effects of age or treatment condition on treatment compliance. There were, however, significant age by group effects by treatment protocol effects. For older patients, the number of days abstinent was greatest and the number of heavy drinking days was fewest among those treated in an individual-focused rather than in a group condition. This study suggested that elderly alcoholics may respond better to individual-focused interventions rather than traditional mixed-age, group-oriented treatment.

Major limitations remain in the treatment compliance literature, including a lack of drinking outcome data, failure to report on treatment drop-outs, and variations in definitions of treatment completion. Few carefully controlled, prospective treatment outcome studies including sufficiently large numbers of older subjects who meet criteria for alcohol dependence have been conducted to address the methodological limitations of prior work.

Prospective Studies of Treatment Outcomes

Few prospective treatment outcome studies have been reported in the literature, in part due to the complexity of studying older adults in treatment and in part due to difficulties in following them after completion of treatment. Thus, sample sizes tend to be too small to provide definitive results. One exception is a study of 137 male veterans (age 45–59 years, $n=64$; age 60–69 years, $n=62$; age 70 years and older, $n=11$) with alcohol problems who were randomly assigned after detoxification to age-specific treatment or standard mixed-age treatment (Kashner et al. 1992). Outcomes at 6 months and 1 year showed that elder-specific program patients were 2.9 times more likely at 6 months, and 2.1 times more likely at 1 year, to report abstinence compared with the mixed-age-group patients. Treatment groups, however, could not be compared at baseline because baseline alcohol consumption and alcohol severity data were not included in the study. A recent prospective comparison of older versus younger adults seeking addiction treatment confirmed prior reports demonstrating greater adherence to treatment in older adults (Oslin et al. 2002). This study also demonstrated that older adults have greater reductions in drinking with higher rates of abstinence and low rates of relapse compared with younger adults.

Limitations of Treatment Outcome Research

Although examination of factors related to program completion is important for identifying the characteristics of patients who will remain in treatment, existing studies have an inherent selectivity bias and provide no information on treatment drop-outs or on short- or long-term treatment outcomes. Other issues with sampling may also limit the generalizability of previous studies. For example, the majority of reports on alcoholism treatment outcome for older adults have included only male subjects, with virtually no studies addressing treatment of prescription or illicit drug use in this population. Furthermore, age cutoffs for inclusion in studies have varied widely, and have included non-elderly individuals in the "older" category, with several studies including individuals as young as age 45. In addition to these issues, most studies have used relatively unstructured techniques for assessing alcohol-related symptoms and consequences of drinking behavior. Finally, the manner in which outcomes have been assessed has been narrow in focus.

Most studies have dichotomized treatment outcome (abstention versus relapse) based solely on drinking behavior. Given evidence from numerous studies that heavy or binge drinking is more strongly related to alcohol consequences than is average alcohol consumption (Anda et al. 1988; Chermack et al. 1996; Kranzler et al. 1990), it is possible important differences exist in outcome for non-abstinent individuals, depending on whether their reuse of alcohol after treatment involves binge drinking. For these reasons, researchers have suggested that non-abstinent drinking outcomes should be categorized along dimensions such as whether these individuals ever drink to the point of intoxication (Heather and Tebbutt 1989). Furthermore, most studies have not addressed other relevant domains that may be positively affected by treatment, such as physical and mental health status and psychological distress.

The development and testing of elder-specific treatment programs as well as further assessment of outcomes for older adults in treatment programs that include younger and older adults need to be further addressed. As mentioned earlier in this chapter, with the aging of the baby-boom generation, new challenges in the treatment of substance use disorders can be anticipated.

Special Issue: Benzodiazepine Withdrawal and Treatment

Addressing inappropriate use and misuse of medications relies on physicians and pharmacists to monitor medication use carefully, avoiding dangerous combinations of drugs, medications with a high potential for side effects, and ineffective or unnecessary medications. A practical approach to monitoring psychoactive medication use would be to reevaluate use every 3–6 months. Only patients with a documented response to the treatment should continue on to maintenance treatment. Patients without a response or with partial response should be reevaluated to consider the appropriate diagnosis and further care. This consideration is also a point in which a consultation with a specialty geriatric mental health provider could be advantageous.

Although withdrawal from benzodiazepines may be considered difficult, Rickels et al. (1991) demonstrated that elderly patients could successfully be withdrawn from chronic benzodiazepine use. However, they also demonstrated that elderly patients are more likely to return to benzodiazepine use within 3 years of discontinuation. Given that the negative effects of benzodiazepines, such as increased risks of falls and cognitive effects, are dose dependent and occur more often with longer acting medications, a practical approach to managing long-term use would be to decrease the medication to the lowest possible dose and avoid long-acting medications.

Once significant substance use and any associated problems have been identified, it is important to note that older persons with substance use problems often present with a variety of treatment needs. It is therefore important to have an array of services available that can be tailored to these individual needs and also to have the flexibility to adapt to changing needs over time. The spectrum of alcohol interventions for older adults ranges from minimal advice or brief structured interventions for at-risk or problem drinkers to formalized alcoholism treatment for drinkers who meet criteria for abuse and/or dependence. The array of formalized treatment options available includes various psychotherapeutic options, educational tools, rehabilitative and residential models, and psychopharmacological treatments. An example of how this tailoring of needs is important is the contrast between the at-risk drinker or benzodiazepine user and the severely dependent patient. It is unlikely that the at-risk user will need services as intense as those used for the severely dependent patient in order to be successful. Indeed, requiring the at-risk drinker to attend a mandatory set of services may be more detrimental than helpful. The use of brief interventions and individual therapy focused on alcohol use can also easily be incorporated into the context of the treatment of depression without necessitating a referral to a specialty addiction service.

Medical and Psychiatric Comorbidities

The consequences of heavy alcohol consumption are discussed in many studies and textbooks. However, there is emerging evidence of medical risks to older adults with alcohol use below the levels that generally require specialized treatment. At-risk alcohol drinking has been demonstrated to increase the risk of strokes caused by bleeding, although it decreases the risk of strokes caused by blocked blood vessels (Hansagi 1995). Non-abusive alcohol use has also been demonstrated to impair driving-related skills even at low levels of consumption, and it may lead to other injuries such as falls (Kivela et al. 1989). Of particular importance to the elderly individual is the potential interaction between alcohol and both prescribed and over-the-counter medications, especially psychoactive medications such as benzodiazepines, barbiturates, and antidepressants. Alcohol is also known to interfere with the metabolism of medications such as digoxin and warfarin (Adams 1995; Fraser 1997; Hylek 1998).

Although the impact of excessive alcohol use on activities of daily living is not fully understood, several studies have demonstrated a relationship between alcohol use and functional abilities, especially among older subjects. Blow et al. (2000) examined the relationship between alcohol use and health functioning in a sample of older adults screened in primary care settings. A total of 8,578 older adults (aged 55–97 years) with regularly scheduled appointments in primary care clinics were screened and categorized based on alcohol consumption levels as abstainers, low-risk drinkers, and at-risk drinkers. There were significant effects of drinking status on the areas of general health, physical functioning, physical role functioning, bodily pain, vitality, mental health, emotional role, and social functioning, controlling for age and gender. Low-risk drinkers scored significantly better than abstainers. At-risk drinkers had significantly poorer mental health functioning than low-risk drinkers. In an earlier study by Ensrud (1994), a prior history of alcohol use had an odds ratio of 2.2 in predicting impairment in activities of daily living among older women. Alcohol use was more strongly correlated with impairment than smoking, age, use of anxiolytics, stroke, or lower grip strength. In contrast to this finding, several authors have demonstrated that among older, community-dwelling persons, moderate alcohol use is associated with fewer falls, greater mobility, and improved physical functioning when compared with a comparison group of non-drinkers (LaCroix 1993; D.E. Nelson et al. 1992; H. Nelson et al. 1994; O'Loughlin et al. 1993). These studies did not include many heavy drinkers or subjects with alcohol use disorders. Together, these studies suggest that alcohol consumption in older persons may exhibit a protective effect in moderate doses similar to the protective effect on cardiovascular morbidity and a detrimental effect with more excessive alcohol use (Scherr et al. 1992).

Comorbid Depression

Epidemiologic studies have clearly demonstrated comorbidity between alcohol use and psychiatric symptoms in adults under age 65. A few studies indicate that a dual diagnosis with alcoholism is an important concern with adults age 65 and older (Blazer and Williams 1980; Blow et al. 1992; Finlayson et al. 1988; Oslin et al. 1999; Saunders et al. 1991).

Comorbid depressive symptoms are not only common in late life but are also an important factor in the course and prognosis of psychiatric disorders. Depressed persons who are alcohol dependent have been shown to have a more complicated clinical course of depression with an increased risk of suicide and more social dysfunction than nondepressed alcoholics (Conwell 1991; Cook 1991). Alcohol abuse prior to later life has also been shown to predict a more severe and chronic course for depression (Cook 1991).

A limited number of studies address the treatment of patients who present with comorbid alcoholism and depression. Rigorous treatment recommendations are scarce, because many patients with comorbid substance use are excluded from clinical trials. For example, concurrent alcohol or drug misuse was found to be the greatest factor for exclusion (17%) of subjects from antidepressant trials. Other significant exclusions included current use of an antidepressant (15%), concurrent physical disability (14%), and organizational difficulty (16%) (Partonen et al. 1996). Several recent studies have included subjects with comorbid major depression and alcoholism. In one study, McGrath et al. (1996) conducted a 12-week placebo-controlled trial of imipramine in outpatients with comorbid major depression and alcoholism. The results demonstrated an antidepressant effect of the medication but no overall effect on drinking outcomes, and less than half of those studies had improvement in both their depression and drinking.

Mason et al. (1996) conducted a placebo-controlled study of desipramine in patients with alcoholism with and without major depression. In this study, subjects with depression had a diagnosis of secondary major depression, and sample size was small, with 10–15 subjects in each group. Despite this, a significant drug effect was found, with reduced depressive symptoms in the desipramine-treated group compared with the placebo-treated group. No effect was found on the number of subjects who relapsed, but there was a significant increase in the time to relapse. In a third study, Cornelius et al. (1996) evaluated subjects with primary major depression and comorbid alcoholism. Patients were randomly assigned to placebo or fluoxetine. Fluoxetine significantly improved depressive symptoms over a period of 12 weeks and reduced total alcohol consumption, although no information was provided regarding the number of subjects who achieved full remission from both illnesses. In a fourth study, Roy-Byrne et al. (2000) examined nefazadone as monotherapy in treating primary depression complicated by alcoholism. This study demonstrated an antidepressant effect but no effect on drinking outcomes.

Published literature on combinations of pharmacological agents, such as naltrexone and an antidepressant, for treatment of major depression and alcoholism is also absent. However, the rationale for treating both disorders is sound and is logically based on the concurrent treatment of any two disorders such as hypertension and major depression or cognitive disorders and major depression. All of the studies using a single pharmacotherapeutic strategy resulted in modest outcomes with significant numbers of patients who remained ill at the end of the study. Thus, these studies are encouraging but suggest the need for an improved treatment regimen and the need to address both depression and alcoholism in patients with concurrent symptoms.

Although these studies have begun to shed light on the treatment of comorbid depression and alcoholism, they have not addressed treatment of older adults. In the absence of empirical data, specific treatment recommendations for older adults with comorbid substance abuse are derived from a consensus development process that reviewed existing data to develop treatment guidelines (Blow 1998).

Suicide

Suicide among the elderly is a tragic and potentially preventable problem. Compared with the general population, rates of suicide are significantly higher for people age 55 and older. Depression and alcohol abuse are the two most common psychiatric diagnoses of older suicide victims. Rates of suicide in this population are projected to increase as the baby-boom generation ages, and alcohol consumption patterns of this generation may further exacerbate this problem. Depression and alcohol abuse are underdetected and undertreated in older populations; thus, improvements in detection and appropriate treatment could lead to prevention of elder suicide.

Suicide ranks among the top 10 leading causes of death in the United States. Suicide was the eighth leading cause of death for all Americans in 1998, with 11.3 completed suicides for every 100,000 people. Among older adults, this rate is 16.9 completed suicides per 100,000. Older adults accounted for 12.7% of the population but committed 19% of the suicides in 1998 (Murphy 2000). Across the life course, men are at greater risk for suicide than women, and whites are at greater risk than nonwhites (Conwell and Brent 1995; Grabbe et al. 1997). In addition, men over age 85 commit suicide at six times the national rate: 65 per 100,000 (Moore et al. 2000).

The role of alcohol abuse in elder suicide is complex. Alcohol abuse is more prevalent among the suicidal elderly than the nonsuicidal. Age-related stresses may exacerbate alcohol use problems. Alcoholism is also associated with depression for the elderly. In studies of elder suicides, substance abuse disorders are evident. Carney et al. (1994) found that 22% of people age 60–88 who had successfully committed suicide had a substance use disorder (solely or in combination with an affective disorder). Among older suicide victims with psychiatric contact prior to death, 13.2 had alcoholism as a primary diagnosis. Rates of diagnosed alcoholism among suicide completers for both sexes vary by age (age 50–55, 7.7%; age 56–63, 18.0%; age 64–73, 1.7%; age 74 and older, 5.8%).

Of those with alcohol in their bloodstreams during a suicide completion, 71% had blood levels of 0.10% or greater. In a large-scale study (N=10,134) comparing deaths of people age 65 or older, suicide completers had higher rates of emotional or mental disorders and more visits to a psychiatrist the year before death and were more likely to be moderate to heavy drinkers than those who died of natural causes or injury (Grabbe et al. 1997). Moderate and heavy alcohol users were approximately nine times more likely to die by suicide than by natural causes or injury.

If alcohol is involved in an elder suicide attempt, the level of alcohol used tends to be high (Conwell and Brent 1995). Furthermore, although 10.5% of older persons attempting suicide received alcohol abuse diagnosis after admission to a psychiatric/

medical facility, only 1% of these were referred to a substance abuse program for treatment. Studies of suicidal ideation, however, have not indicated a relationship between alcohol use or alcohol abuse problems and tendency to suicidal ideation.

Dementia

The relationship between alcohol use and dementing illnesses such as Alzheimer's disease is complex. To differentiate alcohol-related dementia from Alzheimer's disease and to determine whether alcohol use, especially heavy use, influences Alzheimer's disease requires autopsy studies that can establish neuropathologic diagnoses. Although the rates of alcohol-related dementia in late life differ according to the diagnostic criteria used and the nature of the population studied, there is a consensus that alcohol contributes significantly to the acquired cognitive deficits of late life (Robins et al. 1984; Saunders et al. 1991). Among subjects over the age of 55 evaluated in the Epidemiologic Catchment Area study (George et al. 1991), the prevalence of a lifetime history of alcohol abuse or dependence was 1.5 times greater among persons with mild and severe cognitive impairment than those with no cognitive impairment. Sleep disorders and sleep disturbances are also comorbid disorders associated with excessive alcohol use. Alcohol causes well-established changes in sleep patterns such as decreased sleep latency, decreased stage IV sleep, and precipitation or aggravation of sleep apnea (Wagman et al. 1997). In addition, common age-associated changes in sleep can all be worsened by alcohol use and depression. Because these physical and psychiatric comorbidities are of concern when working with older adults, it is helpful to keep potential comorbid factors in mind as part of any general health screening.

Summary

Substance use and abuse in later life is a growing public health issue. As older adults live longer and as generational changes occur, more older adults are abusing alcohol and other substances than ever before. As a complicating factor in the treatment of depression, use or abuse of alcohol, cigarettes, and possibly benzodiazepines represents a significant barrier to positive treatment outcomes. Thus, it seems imperative that mental health providers be able to recognize these issues and make the management of substance use problems a part of the treatment plan for depression.

Because few older adults with substance abuse problems seek help from addiction services, it can be argued that the focus of identification and initial management of addiction problems in late life should be addressed by mental health professionals. All too often, older adults find the maze of insurance paperwork and referrals to be complex, and these logistic issues may severely limit patient access to formal care. This is particularly true of older adults with addiction problems who must cope with these logistic barriers as well as substantial personal barriers in the way of shame and stigma. It is also not clear whether dividing up care between multiple providers, such as a depression specialist and addiction specialist, is beneficial to patients. Because older patients with comorbid depression and substance use are more likely to seek help for their depression, mental health professionals may be particularly poised to manage older patients with comorbid substance abuse. However, all behavioral health providers should be trained in the management of depression and substance abuse.

Conclusions

Brief strategies, including minimal advice, structured brief intervention protocols, and referral to specialized treatment, now exist for use with older adults whose drinking patterns put them at risk for alcohol-related problems. Although progress has been made in understanding the effectiveness of screening, brief interventions, and treatments for older adults, it remains to be determined how these protocols will fit into the broad spectrum of health care settings as a routine part of clinical care; how to target specific interventions/treatments to appropriate subgroups of older adults (e.g., women, minorities); and how to best approach prescription and illicit drug misuse in this population.

Research in the substance abuse field has led to the development of screening, intervention, and referral techniques that are both clinically and cost effective. Changes in the health care environment in the United States underscores the importance of using brief, cost-effective techniques and technologies as part of the spectrum of prevention, interventions, and treatments with the elderly. The use of alcohol screening and interventions targeted to the characteristics of older at-risk drinkers move the field toward providing best practices care to a vulnerable population.

References

Adams WL: Interactions between alcohol and other drugs. Int J Addict 30:1903–1923, 1995

Adams WL, Barry KL, Fleming MF: Screening for problem drinking in older primary care patients. JAMA 276:1964–1967, 1996

American Psychiatric Association: Diagnostic and Statistical Manual of Mental Disorders, Fourth Edition Text Revision. Washington, DC, American Psychiatric Association, 2000

Anda RF, Williamson DF, Remington PL: Alcohol and fatal injuries among U.S. adults: findings from the NHANES I Epidemiologic Follow-up Study. JAMA 260:2529–2532, 1988

Atkinson RM: Aging and alcohol use disorders: diagnostic issues in the elderly. Int Psychogeriatr 2:55–72, 1990

Atkinson RM: Treatment programs for aging alcoholics, in Alcohol and Aging. Edited by Beresford TP, Gomberg ES. New York, Oxford University Press, 1995

Atkinson RM, Tolson RL, Turner JA: Late versus early onset problem drinking in older men. Alcohol Clin Exp Res 14:574–579, 1990

Atkinson RM, Tolson RL, Turner JA: Factors affecting outpatient treatment compliance of older male problem drinkers. J Stud Alcohol 54:102–106, 1993

Babor TF, Ritson EB, Hodgson RJ: Alcohol-related problems in the primary health care setting: a review of early intervention strategies. Br J Addict 81:23–46, 1986

Babor TF, Longabaugh R, Zweben A, et al: Issues in the definition and measurement of drinking outcomes in alcoholism treatment research. J Stud Alcohol Suppl 12:101–111, 1994

Barry KL: Alcohol and drug abuse, in Fundamentals of Clinical Practice: A Textbook On the Patient, Doctor, and Society. Edited by Mengel M, Molleman W. New York, Oxford University Press, 1997

Barry KL: Brief Interventions and Brief Therapies for Substance Abuse (TIPS #34). Rockville, MD, U.S. Department of Health and Human Services, Public Health Service, Substance Abuse and Mental Health Services Administration, Center for Substance Abuse Treatment, 1999

Barry KL, Blow FC: Screening and assessment of alcohol problems in older adults, in Handbook of Assessment in Clinical Gerontology. Edited by Lichtenberg P. New York, Wiley, 1999, pp 243–269

Barry KL, Fleming MF: Computerized administration of alcoholism screening tests in a primary care setting. J Am Board Fam Pract 3:93–98, 1990

Barry KL, Oslin D, Blow FC: Alcohol Problems in Older Adults: Prevention and Management. New York, Springer, 2001

Blazer D, Williams CD: Epidemiology of dysphoria and depression in an elderly population. Am J Psychiatry 137:439–444, 1980

Blow FC: Substance Abuse Among Older Adults (TIP#26). Rockville, MD, U.S. Department of Health and Human Services, Public Health Service, Substance Abuse and Mental Health Services Administration, Center for Substance Abuse Treatment, 1998

Blow FC, Brower KJ, Schulenberg JE, et al: The Michigan Alcoholism Screening Test—Geriatric Version (MAST-G): a new elderly specific screening instrument (abstract). Alcohol Clin Exp Res 16:372, 1992

Blow FC, Walton MA, Barry KL, et al: The relationship between alcohol problems and health functioning of older adults in primary care settings. J Am Geriatr Soc 48:7697–74, 2000

Brower KJ, Mudd S, Blow FC, et al: Severity and treatment of alcohol withdrawal in elderly versus younger patients. Alcohol Clin Exp Res 18:196–201, 1994

Carney SS, Rich CL, Burke PA, et al: Suicide over 60: the San Diego study. J Am Geriatr Soc 42:174–180, 1994

Chermack ST, Blow FC, Hill EM, et al: The relationship between alcohol symptoms and consumption among older drinkers. Alcohol Clin Exp Res 20:1153–1158, 1996

Chick J, Lloyd G, Crombie E: Counseling problem drinkers in medical wards: a controlled study. BMJ 290:965–7, 1985

Conwell Y: Suicide in elderly patients, in Diagnosis and Treatment of Depression in Late Life. Washington, DC, American Psychiatric Press, 1991

Conwell Y, Brent D: Suicide and aging, I: patterns of psychiatric diagnosis. Int Psychogeriatr 7:149–164, 1995

Cook BL, Winokur G, Garvey MJ, et al: Depression and previous alcoholism in the elderly. Br J Psychiatry 158:72–75, 1991

Cornelius JR, Salloum IM, Day NL, et al: Patterns of suicidality and alcohol use in alcoholics with major depression. Alcohol Clin Exp Res 20:1451–5, 1996

Day JC: Population projections of the United States by age, sex, race, and hispanic origin: 1995–2050. Washington, DC, U.S. Bureau of Census, 1996

Doll R, Peto R, Hall E, et al: Mortality in relation to consumption of alcohol: 13 years' observations on male British doctors. BMJ 309:911–918, 1994

Dufour M, Fuller RK: Alcohol in the elderly. Annu Rev Med 46:123–132, 1995

Ensrud K, Nevitt MC, Yunis C, et al: Correlates of impaired function in older women. J Am Geriatr Soc 42:481–489, 1994

Finlayson RE, Hurt RD, Davis LJ Jr, et al: Alcoholism in elderly persons: a study of the psychiatric and psychosocial features of 216 inpatients. Mayo Clin Proc 63:761–768, 1988

Fleming MF, Barry KL (eds): Addictive Disorders: A Practical Guide to Treatment. St. Louis, MO, Mosby Yearbook Medical, 1992

Fleming MF, Barry KL, Manwell LB, et al: Brief physician advice for problem alcohol drinkers: a randomized controlled trial in community-based primary care practices. Alcohol Alcohol 277:1039–1045, 1997

Fleming MF, Manwell LB, Barry KL, et al: Brief physician advice for alcohol problems in older adults: a randomized community-based trial. J Fam Pract 48:378–384, 1999

Foy A, March S, Drinkwater V: Use of an objective clinical scale in the assessment and management of alcohol withdrawal in a large general hospital. Alcohol Clin Exp Res 12:360–364, 1988

Fraser AG: Pharmacokinetic interactions between alcohol and other drugs. Clin Pharmacokinet 33:79–90, 1997

Fuchs VR: Health care for the elderly: how much? Who will pay for it? Health Affairs 18:11–21, 1999

Gambert SR, Katsoyannis KK: Alcohol-related medical disorders of older heavy drinkers, in Alcohol and Aging. Edited by Beresford T, Gomberg E. New York, Oxford University Press, 1995

George L: Cognitive impairment, in Psychiatric Disorders in America: The Epidemiologic Catchment Area Study. Edited by Robins LN, Regier DA. New York, Free Press, 1991, pp 291–327

Grabbe L, Demi A, Camann MA, et al: The health status of elderly persons in the last year of life: a comparison of deaths by suicide, injury, and natural causes. Am J Public Health 87:434–437, 1997

Greist JH, Klein MH, Erdman HP, et al: Comparison of computer- and interviewer-administered versions of the Diagnostic Interview Schedule. Hosp Community Psychiatry 38:1304–1311, 1987

Gurland BJ, Cross PS: Epidemiology of psychopathology in old age: some implications for clinical services. Psychiatr Clin North Am 5:11–26, 1982

Hansagi H, Romelsjo A, Gerhardsson de Verdier M, et al: Alcohol consumption and stroke mortality: 20-year follow up of 15077 men and women. Stroke 26:1768–1773, 1995

Heather N, Tebbutt J: Definitions of non-abstinent and abstinent categories in alcoholism treatment outcome classifications: a review and proposal. Drug Alcohol Depend 24:83–93, 1989

Hylek E, Heiman H, Skates SJ, et al: Acetaminophen and other risk factors for excessive warfarin anticoagulation. JAMA 279:657–662, 1998

Institute of Medicine: Assessment in Broadening the Base of Treatment for Alcohol Problems. Washington, DC, National Academy Press, 1990

Kashner TM, Rodell DE, Ogden SR, et al: Outcomes and costs of two VA inpatient treatment programs for older alcoholic patients. Hosp Community Psychiatry 43:985–989, 1992

Kivela SL, Nissinen A, Ketola A: Alcohol consumption and mortality in aging or aged Finnish men. J Clin Epidemiol 42:61–68, 1989

Klatsky AL, Armstrong MA, Friedman GD: Red wine, white wine, liquor, beer, and risk for coronary artery disease hospitalization. Am J Cardiol 80:416–420, 1997

Kranzler HR, Babor TF, Lauerman RJ: Problems associated with average alcohol consumption and frequency of intoxication in a medical population. Alcohol Clin Exp Res 14:119–126, 1990

Kristenson H, Ohlin H, Hulten-Nosslin M-B, et al: Identification and intervention of heavy drinking in middle-aged men: results and follow-up of 24–60 months of long-term study with randomized controls. Alcohol Clin Exp Res 7:203–209, 1983

Krop JS, Powe NR, Weller WE, et al: Patterns of expenditures and use of services among older adults with diabetes: implications for the transition to capitated managed care. Diabetes Care 21:747–752, 1998

LaCroix AZ, Guralnik JM, Berkman LF, et al: Maintaining mobility in late life. Am J Epidemiol 137:858–869, 1993

Liberto JG, Oslin DW, Ruskin PE: Alcoholism in older persons: a review of the literature. Hosp Community Psychiatry 43:975–984, 1992

Maixner SM, Mellow AM, Tandon R: The efficacy, safety, and tolerability of antipsychotics in the elderly. J Clin Psychiatry 60(suppl 8):29–41, 1999

Mason BJ, Kocsis JH, Ritvo EC, et al: A double-blind, placebo-controlled trial of desipramine for primary alcohol dependence stratified on the presence or absence of major depression. JAMA 275:761–767, 1996

McGrath PJ, Nunes EV, Stewart JW, et al: Imipramine treatment of alcoholics with primary depression: a placebo-controlled clinical trial. Arch Gen Psychiatry 53:232–240, 1996

Miller WR, Hester RK: Treating Addictive Behaviors: Processes of Change. New York, Plenum, 1986

Miller WR, Munoz RF: How to Control Your Drinking. Englewood Cliffs, NJ, Prentice-Hall, 1976

Miller WR, Rollnick S: Motivational Interviewing: Preparing People to Change Addictive Behavior, 2nd Edition. New York, Guilford, 2002

Miller WR, Taylor CA: Relative effectiveness of bibliotherapy, individual and group self-control training in the treatment of problem drinkers. Addict Behav 5:13–24, 1980

Moore AA, Hays RD, Reuben DB, et al: Using a criterion standard to validate the Alcohol-Related Problems Survey (ARPS): a screening measure to identify harmful and hazardous drinking in older persons. Aging (Milano) 12:221–227, 2000

Murphy SL: National Vital Statistics report: Deaths—final data for 1998. Washington, DC, National Center for Health Statistics, 2000

National Institute on Alcohol Abuse and Alcoholism: Diagnostic criteria for alcohol abuse. Alcohol Alert 30:1–6, 1995

Nelson DE, Sattin RW, Langlois JA, et al: Alcohol as a risk factor for fall injury events among elderly persons living in the community. J Am Geriatr Soc 40:658–661, 1992

Nelson H, Stone KL, Cummings SR, et al: Smoking, alcohol, and neuromuscular and physical function of older women. JAMA 272:1825–1831, 1994

O'Loughlin JL, Robitaille Y, Boivin J-F, et al: Incidence of and risk factors for falls and injurious falls among the community-dwelling elderly. Am J Epidemiol 137:342–354, 1993

Oslin DW, O'Brien CP, Katz IR: The disabling nature of comorbid depression among older DUI recipients. Am J Addict 8:128–135, 1999

Oslin DW, Pettinati HP, Volpicelli JR: Alcoholism treatment adherence: older age predicts better adherence and drinking outcomes. Am J Geriatr Psychiatry 10:740–747, 2002

Partonen T, Sihvo S, Lonnqvist JK: Patients excluded from an antidepressant efficacy trial. J Clin Psychiatry 57:572–575, 1996

Persson J, Magnusson PH: Early intervention in patients with excessive consumption of alcohol: a controlled study. Alcohol 6:403–408, 1989

Poikolainen K: Epidemiologic assessment of population risks and benefits of alcohol use. Alcohol Alcohol Suppl 1:27–34, 1991

Rice C, Longabaugh R, Beattie M, et al: Age group differences in response to treatment for problematic alcohol use. Addiction 88:1369–1375, 1993

Rickels K, Case WG, Schweizer E, et al: Long-term benzodiazepine users 3 years after participation in a discontinuation program. Am J Psychiatry 148:757–761, 1991

Robins LN, Helzer JE, Weissman MM, et al: Lifetime prevalence of specific psychiatric disorders in three sites. Arch Gen Psychiatry 41:949–958, 1984

Roy-Byrne PP, Pages KP, Russo JE, et al: Nefazodone treatment of major depression in alcohol-dependent patients: a double-blind, placebo-controlled trial. J Clin Psychopharmacol 20:129–136, 2000

Saunders PA, Copeland JRM, Dewey ME, et al: Heavy drinking as a risk factor for depression and dementia in elderly men. Br J Psychiatry 159:213–216, 1991

Scherr PA, LaCroix AZ, Wallace RB, et al: Light to moderate alcohol consumption and mortality in the elderly. J Am Geriatr Soc 40:651–657, 1992

Schneider EL, Guralnik JM: The aging of America: impact on health care costs. JAMA 263:2335–2340, 1990

Schonfeld L, Dupree LW: Antecedents of drinking for early and late-onset elderly alcohol abusers. J Stud Alcohol 52:587–592, 1991

Schuckit MA, Pastor PA Jr: The elderly as a unique population: alcoholism. Alcohol Clin Exp Res 2:31–38, 1978

Sullivan JT, Sykora K, Schneiderman J, et al: Assessment of alcohol withdrawal: the revised clinical institute withdrawal assessment for alcohol scale (CIWA-Ar). Br J Addict 84:1353–1357, 1989

Wagman AM, Allen RP, Upright D: Effects of alcohol consumption upon parameters of ultradian sleep rhythms in alcoholics. Adv Exp Med Biol 85A:601–616, 1997

Waldo DR, Sonnefeld ST, McKusick DR, et al: Health expeditures by age group, 1977 and 1987. Health Care Financ Rev 10:111–120, 1989

Wetle T: Living longer, aging better: aging research comes of age. JAMA 278:1376–1377, 1997

Wiens AN, Menustik CE, Miller SI, et al: Medical-behavioral treatment of the older alcoholic patient. Am J Drug Alcohol Abuse 9:461–475, 1982

Chapter 5

Geriatric Psychiatry at the Crossroads of Public Policy and Clinical Practice

Christopher C. Colenda, M.D, M.P.H.
Stephen J. Bartels, M.D., M.S.
Joel E. Streim, M.D.
Christine deVries

Overview: Scope of the Burden of Mental Illness in Late Life and Future Service Demand

From a public policy perspective, few chronic illnesses have higher disease burden for older Americans than do late-life mental disorders. Recently revised prevalence estimates using modified "clinically significant criteria" from the original Epidemiologic Catchment Area (ECA) data suggest that between 14.2% and 17.3% of adults over age 55 have a "clinically significant mental or substance abuse disorder" (Narrow et al. 2002; Regier et al. 1984). The addition of the "clinical significance" criterion to prevalence estimates (e.g., symptoms were such that the respondent mentioned them to a doctor, took medication for them, or they interfered with the respondent's everyday life) reduced previous ECA estimates between 28% and 40%, depending on the point estimate used. The precision of combining recent census data with the revised prevalence rate information is imperfect at best; however, when the data are combined, between 8.4 and 10.3 million individuals over age 55, or about 5–6 million individuals over age 65, may have clinically significant mental disorders

(Narrow et al. 2002; U.S. Census Bureau 2001). Most of these individuals have anxiety disorders (10.6%–11.4%), followed by mood disorders (3.4%), severe cognitive disorders (2.0%–2.1%), and alcohol use disorders (2.0%–2.6%) (Narrow et al. 2002). Less prevalent are schizophrenia and schizophreniform disorders (0.4%) and bipolar I and bipolar II disorders (0.1% each).

Using these prevalence estimates to forecast future rates, it is conceivable that by 2020, when a substantial portion of the baby-boom generation surpasses age 65 years (about 53 million people) (U.S. Census Bureau 1996), between 7.5 and 9.2 million individuals could experience mental illness in late life.

This chapter reviews current facets of the mental health service delivery system for older adults in the United States. We concentrate on the following: a) current trends in federal expenditures for health care and mental health care, b) trends in Medicare managed care enrollments, c) regulatory trends in long term care, d) special concerns for older adults with severe mental illness, and e) current legislative and executive policy initiatives.

The United States is far from creating an integrated longitudinal continuum of mental health care for the elderly. Our system of care for mental disorders in late life remains fragmented, inextricably linked to primary care, complicated by medical-psychiatric co-morbidity, under funded, and plagued by irrational incentives and access barriers (Colenda et al. 2002; Fogel 1994). That said, as we enter an era that will test the capacity of the system to deliver high-quality, state-of-the-art, and compassionate care, it is important to understand the characteristics of the current system that, in turn, can shape future health services innovations. What we hope to avoid is a failed experiment in social Darwinism that jeopardizes the well-being of the nation's most vulnerable population.

Trends in Health Expenditures: "Form and Finance"

National Health Expenditures

During the 1990s, federal and state policymakers were far more concerned with managing health care costs than with designing integrated systems of care. The United States has struggled with the need to slow the growth of rising medical expenditures. For example, in 1980, national health expenditures approximated $246 billion or about 8.8% of the gross domestic product (GNP). In 1990 these expenditures increased to about $696 billion, or about 13.4% of the GNP. During the 1990s, with the combination of an expanding GNP and managed care cost containment, national health expenditures dropped to 13.0% of the GNP by 1999 despite overall expenditures increasing to $1.2 trillion (Figure 5–1). By 2001, however, medical inflation began to increase. National health expenditures increased to 13.4% of the GNP, or $1.4 trillion. Given current expenditure and population trends, the Centers for Medicare and Medicaid Services (CMS) estimate that by 2010 national health expenditures will be 15.9% of the GNP or about $2.6 trillion, nearly double the dollars spent in 2001 (Centers for Medicare and Medicaid Services 2001).

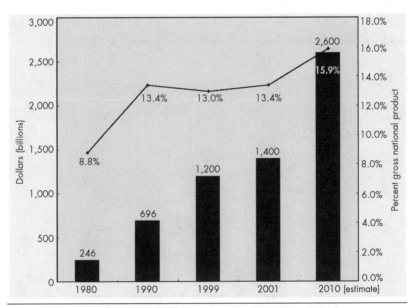

Figure 5–1. National health expenditures (in billions) and as a percent of the gross national product.
Source. Adapted from Centers for Medicare and Medicaid Services 2001, Table 1.

Trends in Medicare Expenditures

Medicare is an important payor of health care services in the United States. In 1980, total Medicare expenditures approximated $37.4 billion or about 15.2% of national health expenditures. In 2000, Medicare expenditures were $224 billion or about 17% of overall health care spending, growing by 5.6% from 1999. CMS estimates that by 2010, Medicare will spend approximately $441 billion and will remain relatively stable at about 16.7% of overall health care spending. The estimated annual rate of increase will hover around 7.0% per year during the 2000–2010 decade (Figure 5–2). Expenditure projections are fraught with uncertainties associated with macroeconomic forecasting. What appears clear, however, are the market forces that will affect health expenditures in both the public and private sectors. These include increased spending for prescription drugs due to greater demand created by direct-to-consumer marketing, development of newer therapies with high-cost branded drugs, expanded drug benefit coverage, rising provider and hospital costs, new technology applications, and insurers' inability to negotiate discounts (Levit et al. 2002).

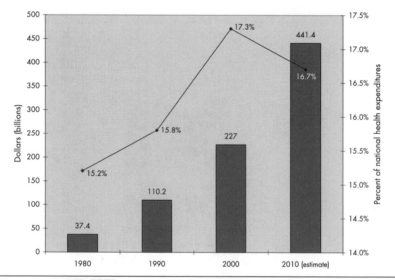

Figure 5–2. Medicare expenditures (in billions) and as a percent of national health expenditures.

Source. Adapted from Centers for Medicare and Medicaid Services 2001, Table 3.

National Mental Health Expenditures

Health insurance coverage for the treatment of mental disorders is typically less generous than for other medical conditions, and the government plays a larger role in financing (U.S. Surgeon General 1999b). Our best estimates of mental health expenditures come from 1996 data. That year, the nation spent more than $99 billion for direct treatment of mental disorders across the life span, or between 9.5% and 10.5% of total health expenditures depending on the data source (Mark et al. 1998; U.S. Surgeon General 1999b). Approximately $69 billion was spent on mental disorders, $18 billion on Alzheimer's disease and dementias, and about $13 billion on addictive disorders. Approximately 53% of all mental health expenditures were paid by the public sector payors, 14% by Medicare, 19% by Medicaid, 18% by other state and local agencies, and 2% by other federal sources. About 27% of mental health coverage was paid by private insurance, and 17% was paid "out of pocket" by consumers (U.S. Surgeon General 1999b).

Mental Health Expenditures for Medicare

The proportion of Medicare expenditures devoted to mental health is actually quite small. For example, based on calculations from published government reports, Medicare spent about $9.8 billion for mental health services, or about 4.9% of total Medicare budget in 1996 (U.S. Surgeon General 1999b) (Figure 5–3). The $9.8 billion expended in 1996 was up from just under $5.1 billion in 1994 (Witkin et al. 1998). Most Medicare mental health expenditures went for Part A or hospital-based services. In 1995, Medicare beneficiaries over age 65 years with a primary psychiatric diagnosis accounted for 325,000 hospital and skilled nursing facility stays or 53% of all acute psychiatric payments made by Medicare. The majority of admissions were to psychiatric units in general hospitals (42%), followed by general hospital admissions (29%), psychiatric hospitals (15%), and skilled nursing facilities (14%) (Cano et al. 1997).

In 1998, the Department of Health and Human Services' Office of the Inspector General estimated that Medicare spent about

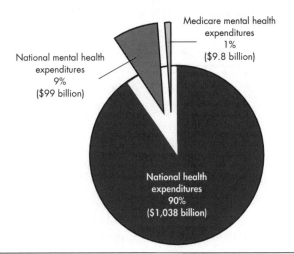

National mental health
expenditures
9%
($99 billion)

Medicare mental health
expenditures
1%
($9.8 billion)

National health
expenditures
90%
($1,038 billion)

Figure 5–3.   Mental health expenditures as a percent of national health expenditures: 1996.
Source.   Data from Centers for Medicare and Medicaid Services 2001, Table 3, and U.S. Surgeon General 1999c.

$1.2 billion for Part B provider services (about 0.6% of total Medicare expenditures), of which $718 million were in outpatient settings (0.3% of total Medicare expenditures) (Office of the Inspector General 2001a). This percentage has remained remarkably stable over the decade despite expanded benefit coverage for outpatient services (Shea 1998; Sherman 1992).

From a policy perspective, why are these data important to understand? First, a comparison of the overall prevalence of clinically significant late-life mental disorders (14%–17%) with the proportion of Medicare expenditures for mental and substance abuse disorders (4.9% of Medicare's budget in 1996) illustrates a striking asymmetry between disease burden and treatment expenditures. Second, underutilization of outpatient services is problematic. Although we do not have good data on geriatric patients, we believe that only about 8% of adults in the general population will receive outpatient mental health treatment, despite the fact that 28% of adults have a diagnosable illness. Thus, 20% of all adults with a diagnosable mental disorder do not receive outpatient treatment during any given year (U.S. Surgeon General 1999b). Third, we know that most older adults initially access mental health treatments and have preferences for receiving mental health treatment through the general medical sector (Marino et al. 1995; Mickus et al. 2002; Regier et al. 1993). Given the cultural stigma of mental illness in our society, which is heightened among older adults, creating integrated systems of care makes intuitive sense. Unfortunately, we do not have good data on the effectiveness of "vertical" (across different health care sectors) or "horizontal" (longitudinal) integration of care (Borson et al. 2001). Finally, federal health care policy that encourages Medicare beneficiaries to enroll in Medicare managed care plans that use commercial approaches to behavioral health management, coupled with concerns over medical inflation, may make integration more difficult to achieve. As we move through this decade, much research is needed to improve actuarial estimates, perceived need, utilization projections, and feasibility studies to test integrated models of care using both cost and quality outcomes.

Overview of Medicare: Circa 2002

The Medicare program covers 95% of the nation's elderly, with expenditures close to $227 billion. Medicare's nearly universal coverage for the elderly is important because of the impact of adverse risk selection on insurance premium costs. Because 11% of the elderly live in poverty and another 6.4% are between poverty and 125% of the poverty level, the actuarial risk for high medical service utilization among the elderly would make private insurance premiums prohibitively high (Medicare Payment Advisory Commission 1999a).

Medicare is composed of three parts: Part A (hospital insurance), Part B (medical insurance), and Part C (Medicare + Choice). Parts A and B, or traditional Medicare, contain features typical of indemnity-like insurance products such as fee-for-service (FFS) payment, deductibles, and coinsurance, but do not have limits on annual personal spending. Part C is a managed care program offered by private companies that was established by the Balanced Budget Act of 1997 (BBA-97; Public Law 105–33) (Centers for Medicare and Medicaid Services 2002).

Traditional Medicare: Parts A and B

Traditional Medicare does not fully cover medical equipment costs and fails to cover prescription medicines and the costs of long-term care. Cost sharing and uncovered benefits have created the private "supplemental insurance" or "medigap" market, the premiums for which constitute the largest source of personal spending for community-dwelling beneficiaries (Medicare Payment Advisory Commission 1999b). Supplemental policies may have inpatient and outpatient mental health benefits, but they are almost universally subject to coverage limits typically found in the commercial market.

With regard to mental health benefits, traditional FFS Medicare includes inpatient psychiatric hospital care (up to 190 days lifetime maximum in free-standing psychiatric hospitals, which is exempt for inpatient psychiatric units in general hospitals) and partial hospitalization. Part B covers medically necessary psychotherapy services provided by psychiatrists, nonpsychiatric physicians, psychologists, and other mental health providers. These services are subject to a 50% copayment, whereas medical management services are subject to a 20% copayment (Centers for Medicare and Medicaid Services 2002).

Medicare + Choice: Part C

Several managed care options existed for Medicare patients prior to the BBA-97, but that 1997 legislation encouraged expansion and diversification of offerings. Prior to 1997, Medicare managed care products included Medicare Risk Contracting (MRC) plans, Point of Service (POS) options, Social health maintenance organizations (HMOs), or demonstration projects called Programs of All-Inclusive Care for the Elderly (PACE). The latter two programs were demonstration projects that combined Medicare and Medicaid funding into one funding base, providing a continuum of health care services including inpatient, outpatient, and long-term care settings (Colenda et al. 2002). Part C expanded managed care options to include medical savings accounts, POS options allowing patients to select from a broader panel of practitioners outside of the HMO network, religious fraternal benefits plans, and other coordinated care plans that meet the Medicare + Choice standards (Medicare Payment Advisory Commission 1999c).

At its peak, about 6.35 million Medicare beneficiaries were enrolled in one of 309 health plans participating in Medicare + Choice, or about 16.4% of all beneficiaries (American Association of Health Plans 2000; Centers for Medicaid and Medicare Services 2003) (Figure 5–4). The enrollment growth slowed significantly from the mid to late 1990s, and beginning in 1999, many managed care companies began to withdraw from the market because of payment rates and regulatory burdens (Medicare Payment Advisory Commission 1999c). Although initial predictions are that a large proportion of Medicare beneficiaries will choose managed care programs because of benefit enticements such as covering pharmacy costs, yearly health screenings, or optical benefits (Langwell et al. 1999), enrollment has continued to decline. By 2002 enrollment dropped to 5.2 million beneficiaries and only 157 participating health plans (Medicare Program 2002).

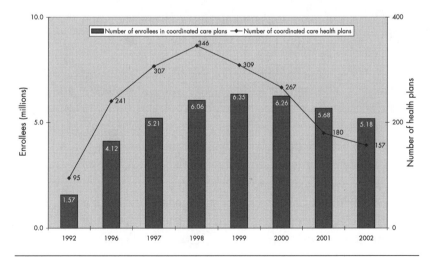

Figure 5–4. Trends in Medicare managed care in the United States, 1992–2000 (all data from December 1 of that year).
Source. Adapted from Centers for Medicare and Medicaid Services 2003.

Mental Health Benefits in Medicare + Choice

With regard to mental health benefits, most MRC plans "carve out" the mental health benefit package, similar to what they do for commercial patient populations. Benefits of such an approach include reduction of HMO staffing and space needs, improved patient confidentiality, and mental health professional input for difficult cases. Proponents note that carve-out financing for mental health services is superior because vendors are able to manage costs and services through superior technical knowledge, skills, and service delivery networks (Bartels and Colenda 1998).

Mental health carve-outs have unique challenges for the elderly, however. Policy issues include definitions of medical necessity criteria, copayment policies, credentialing standards for providers, hospital network standards, rules over geographic access, referral mechanisms, case management guidelines, coordinated mental health and general health care standards, and quality improvement mechanisms (Wells et al. 1995). Actuarial problems include risk adjustment for chronicity and medical-psychiatric comorbidity of late-life mental disorders such as Alzheimer's disease or recurrent major depression (Bartels and Colenda 1998). Carve-out arrangements also pose problems for demonstrating cost offset for mental health services, especially for those patients with significant medical-psychiatric comorbidity (Bartels et al. 1999).

"Carve-in" models also have potential advantages and disadvantages. This benefit design better integrates mental and physical care, decreases access barriers due to stigma, and produces cost offsets in general health care expenditures because of the high medical-psychiatric comorbidity among older adults (Bartels et al. 1999). Other benefits include better collaboration among psychiatric and physical health providers as well as improved psychiatric services for those older patients who receive most of their mental health service from primary care providers (Mechanic 1997; Mollica and Riley 1996). However, functional integration of mental and general health services are far from guaranteed, and mental health services are likely to receive low priority in these types of managed care arrangements. Comprehensive services for mental health (e.g., parity) may not occur, and payment methodology that adequately risk adjusts for the more seriously ill patients is not well developed, thus placing health plans at risk for substantial financial loss (Bartels et al. 1999; Frank et al. 1997).

The Long Road Toward Mental Health Parity in Medicare

Medicare reimbursement policies for mental health services, especially outpatient services, have been characterized by significant cost sharing by beneficiaries since 1965. Until the reforms that began in the 1980s, Medicare payment policies favored acute inpatient services over outpatient services (Bartels and Colenda 1998). For example, in 2000, Medicare paid inpatient care up to 90 days in a benefit period, paying all but a 1-day deductible of $768 for the first 60 days, and all but $192 for days 61–90 (Health Care Financing Administration 2000b). Beneficiaries also had a 60-day lifetime reserve if hospitalized beyond 90 days, and for each lifetime reserve day, Medicare paid all covered costs except for a daily co-insurance of $388. These amounts changed on a yearly basis, and beneficiaries paid little out-of-pocket expense because their supplemental policies paid the co-payments (Frank 2000).

Conversely, between 1966 and 1988, Medicare covered outpatient mental health services up to a maximum of $500, subject to a 50% copayment—i.e., Medicare only paid $250. In 1984, limitations on medically based psychiatric services for Alzheimer's disease were not subject to the $500 and 50% cap. The Omnibus Budget Reconciliation Acts of 1987 and 1989 (OBRA-87 and OBRA-89, respectively) changed reimbursement for outpatient psychotherapy services. OBRA-87 raised the $500 cap for psychotherapy reimbursement to $2,200, but retained the 50% copayment, effectively paying only $1,100. OBRA-87 exempted medical management of psychotropic medications from the limit in addition to reducing the copayment to 20%. Partial hospitalization services were allowed reimbursement at a rate of 2 days of partial hospitalization for 1 day of inpatient care. OBRA-89 removed the cap on outpatient mental health services, although the 50% copayment was retained (Bartels and Colenda 1998).

Medicare Reform

Medicare reform is an important issue for both health providers and elderly health care consumers. Over the past several years, reform has focused on two broad areas: 1) payment for health services and 2) modification of benefit design. Reform has been modest at best. For example, legislation to simplify the regulatory process as well as provide educational and technical assistance to health care providers has been passed by the U.S. House of Representatives but not by the Senate. Efforts to end the historic discrimination against Medicare beneficiaries seeking outpatient treatment for mental illness or to eliminate the 190-day lifetime cap on inpatient services in psychiatric hospitals have been made, but to date no action has been taken by Congress.

Social Experiments at the State Level: Medicaid Financing and Long-Term Care

Along with Medicare, Medicaid was created with the passage of the Amendments to the Social Security Act of 1965. Medicaid is a joint federal and state program that pays for long-term care in nursing homes and acute care services for the poor. Federal matching rates vary between 50% for the wealthiest states to about 70% for poor states (Frank 2000). Over the years, states have lobbied for and received considerable leeway in defining both eligibility for and the benefit structure of Medicaid (Bartels et al. 1999). Common to Medicaid programs, however, is the 20%–30% reduction in reimbursement schedules compared with regional market rates, in part due to regulations that do not allow costs to be contained by patient cost-sharing mechanisms (Bartels et al. 1999; Frank 2000).

Medicaid expenditures in 1980 were estimated to be about $26 billion. By 2000, they exceeded $201 billion and by 2010 they are projected to be about $446 billion (see Figure 5–1). During this same period, nursing home and home health care increased from $20.1 billion in 1980 to nearly $133 billion in 2000 to a projected $270 billion in 2010 (see Figure 5–2). Medicaid covers about 68% of nursing home residents and over 59% of nursing home costs

(Streim et al. 2002). Of note, the ratio of nursing home expenditures to home health expenditures during the past 20 years has shifted impressively, going from about 7:1 in 1980 to just under 3:1 in 2000. If projections hold, this ratio will drop to about 2:1 by 2010 (Figure 5–5). Thus, although the total amount of long-term care expenditures continues to escalate, an ever-increasing proportion is and will be spent in home-based care, by both legislative and regulatory design and intent of those receiving care.

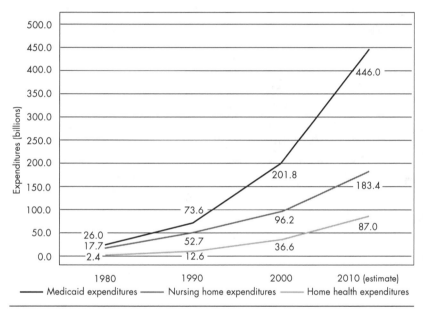

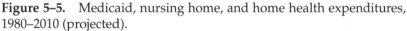

Figure 5–5. Medicaid, nursing home, and home health expenditures, 1980–2010 (projected).
Source. Adapted from Centers for Medicare and Medicaid Services 2001, Tables 2 and 3.

Medicaid and Mental Health Services

It is virtually impossible to determine the proportion of Medicaid mental health dollars spent just on the elderly (Witkin et al. 1998). Most Medicaid expenditures for this group are spent on long-term care services. For example, in 1997 approximately $10,129 per elderly beneficiary was expended; about 75% of this amount was for long-term care services (Physician Payment Review Commission

1997). Despite its limitations, Medicaid covers a broad array of mental health services for adults, and because of joint federal-state matching, strong incentives were created for states to get out of the direct service delivery and evolve into payor and regulator roles (Frank 2000).

Early on, Medicaid recipients were free to choose their providers. However, few providers would accept the low reimbursement rates. More recently, encouraged by federal policy and health care cost reductions observed in the commercial markets, states have implemented Medicaid managed care programs that have been expanded by Medicaid waiver programs, Section 1915(b) and Section 1115 of the Social Security Act. Section 1915(b) allows states to mandate enrollment into managed care programs. Section 1115(a) allows time-limited demonstration projects that test and evaluate innovative approaches to delivery and financing of health care. Section 1115(a) has allowed some states to expand Medicaid eligibility for acute care services, but by and large, it has been used to enroll Medicaid beneficiaries into prepaid managed care programs. How these waiver programs will affect access to mental health or long-term care services by elders has yet to be determined, but as of 1996, about 38.6% of all Medicaid beneficiaries were under Medicaid managed care arrangement, an increase of 12% between 1995 and 1996 (Physician Payment Review Commission 1997).

Mental Health Services in Long-Term Care Settings

Over the past 16 years federal regulations, survey and inspection programs, and payment policy have presented shifting—and often conflicting—incentives and disincentives for the provision of mental health services in nursing homes (Streim et al. 2002).

Beginning with the 1986 Institute of Medicine (IOM) report on improving the quality of care in nursing homes, the need for improved access and quality of mental health services in long-term care has received considerable attention. The 1986 report not only cited the inappropriate use of antipsychotic drugs and physical restraints, but also emphasized the inadequate treatment of depression in U.S. nursing homes (Institute of Medicine, Committee on Nursing Home Regulation 1986). This report served as the cornerstone for the comprehensive Nursing Home Reform Act as part of OBRA '87. It directed the then Health Care Financing Administration (HCFA) to take steps to ensure that unmet mental health needs of nursing home residents were addressed. Regulations require preadmission screening and annual resident review (PASARR) to determine whether patients have mental illness, whether they need active psychiatric treatment, whether they need the level of nursing care provided by a nursing home, and whether the nursing facility can provide the needed mental health services (Health Care Financing Administration 1992a). These regulations were intended to make sure that patients with mental disorders were not placed in nursing homes if there was a need for acute psychiatric treatment (Health Care Financing Administration 1991). Additional regulations required periodic clinical evaluation of nursing home residents using a standardized resident assessment instrument that focused on detection and treatment of newly discovered mental and behavioral symptoms and related functional disability (Health Care Financing Administration 1992b). Together, these regulations provided a clear federal mandate for detection and treatment of mental illness in nursing homes (Streim et al. 2002).

After implementation of these federal regulations, several studies found evidence of a substantial impact on behavioral and psychiatric treatment (Avorn et al. 1992; Rovner et al. 1992; Shorr et al. 1994; Seigler et al. 1997). Regulations that prohibit the use of drugs as chemical restraints and required periodic attempts to taper or discontinue antipsychotic drugs were followed by substantial reductions in the prevalence of antipsychotic drug use. However, a retrospective study in a single nursing facility revealed that 20% of residents whose antipsychotic drug was discontinued or reduced in dose subsequently had the agent resumed or its dose increased (Semla et al. 1994). A more recent study of pharmacy records in eight nursing homes found that of the 17.7% of residents receiving antipsychotic medications, 70.9% had a HCFA-approved diagnostic indication, 90.4% had documentation of appropriate target symptoms, and 90.1% were receiving dosages within the limits specified in the HCFA guidelines (Llorente et al. 1998). Important quality-of-care outcome measures are not found in these studies, such as examining regulatory compliance in relationship to symptom control, functional status, quality of life, and other outcome measures relevant to patient health and well-being (Streim et al. 2002).

Despite statutory and regulatory requirements, there is evidence that a substantial proportion of residents still have undetected psychiatric symptoms and that others do not receive the care they require. Borson et al. (1997) found that 88% of a sample of nursing home residents referred for PASARR screening were appropriately placed based on their care needs but that 55% had unmet mental health services needs and 25% had a psychiatric disorder associated with dementia or mental retardation. Of note, the PASARR exempts patients with dementia from evaluation for the presence of psychiatric illness; permitting nursing home admission regardless of their need for behavioral health care. This is one of the reasons that researchers and clinicians have questioned the utility of the PASARR (Colenda et al. 1999; Snowden and Roy-Byrne 1998).

Many factors contribute to the lack of access and inadequate provision of mental health services in long-term care settings. The most recent IOM report (Institute of Medicine, Committee on Improving Quality in Long-Term Care 2001), however, noted that payment policy and reimbursement mechanisms contain significant disincentives for provision of mental health care. First, the BBA-97 repealed federal standards for reimbursing nursing home care under the Medicaid program. This measure gave states freedom in setting payment rates and promptly resulted in significant disparities across states. For example, the average Medicaid nursing home reimbursement rates in 1998 ranged from a low of $62.58 per day in Nebraska to a high of $329.62 per day in Alaska. Second, BBA-97 altered reimbursement methods for nursing homes that resulted in large budget savings for Medicare. The report identified both measures as "troubling" because they have resulted in the overall withdrawal of substantial resources from long-term care at a time when IOM recommendations require more, not less, funding (Institute of

Medicine, Committee on Improving Quality in Long-Term Care 2001).

A third change occurred in 1999. Social work services were required to be furnished as one of many services "bundled" together under payments made directly to nursing facilities. Thus, psychiatric services provided by nursing home social workers were no longer billable. For nursing homes facing constrained resources and reduced reimbursement in the face of competing regulatory requirements, these changes have the potential to seriously limit the provision of necessary services to maintain the "psychosocial well-being" of nursing home residents (Streim et al. 2002). This is a prime example of contradiction across policy domains: regulatory policy requires mental health assessment and treatment, whereas payment policy undermines this goal by allowing states to underfund nursing homes (Streim et al. 2002).

Monitoring Mental Health Services in Long-Term Care Settings: Recent Surveys by the Office of the Inspector General of the Department of Health and Human Services

The Office of the Inspector General (OIG) of the Department of Health and Human Services (DHHS) has statutory authority to oversee the provision of mental health services to nursing home residents through a nationwide program of audits, investigations, inspections, sanctions, and fraud alerts (Streim et al. 2002). In response to directives from Congress, DHHS, or HCFA, or as part of the OIG's own work agenda, the OIG may assess the appropriateness of services or evaluate quality of care and develop strategies to improve how HCFA pays for and monitors mental health services.

The OIG has conducted two studies on mental health services provided in nursing homes. The first study, released in May 1996 (Office of the Inspector General 1996), was part of a DHHS antifraud initiative called Operation Restore Trust. It was prompted by concern that Medicare was being billed for unnecessary or inappropriate services as observed in the context of 1) increasing numbers of nursing home residents being identified as having mental disorders, 2) expanded Medicare Part B coverage to pay for psychologists and social worker services, and 3) tripling of Medicare mental health expenditures in nursing homes. The study found that 32% of these services were medically unnecessary (e.g., the patient's condition did not warrant the treatment or the patient was unable to benefit from treatment) and 15% were "questionable" (i.e., there were serious questions about the medical necessity of treatment, but insufficient evidence in the medical record to make a clear determination). The report also identified a lack of carrier policies and processes specific to nursing homes and recommended the development of carrier guidelines and screens, the provision of educational activities to mental health service providers, and the conducting of focused medical reviews to limit HCFA's vulnerabilities (Streim et al. 2002).

The second study was released in January 2001 and evaluated the appropriateness of Medicare Part B payments for psychiatric services (Office of the Inspector General 2001b). The study found that 27% of services billed under five psychiatric treatment codes were deemed to be medically unnecessary, based in most cases on a determination that the patient's advance cognitive decline made treatment inappropriate or that the frequency and/or duration of the service was excessive. Similar to the first study, the follow-up investigation found that psychological testing, provided mostly by clinical psychologists, was the service most often found to be medically unnecessary. Least problematic was individual psychotherapy with medical evaluation and management. Compared with the 1996 study, there were more carrier policies that addressed nursing home psychiatric services; however, utilization guidelines remained inconsistent and unclear (Streim et al. 2002).

Although inappropriate diagnostic testing or service delivery is never condoned, the current state of affairs in long-term care has contradictory regulatory assessment and treatment policies that collide with practice and payment. The OIG has recommended that the CMS work with carriers to develop guidelines for appropriate frequency and duration of the psychiatric services reviewed, including psychological testing, and encourage providers to furnish more thorough documentation of mental health services (Streim et al. 2002).

Mental Health Policy for Older Adults With Severe Mental Illness

At least 1% of individuals over age 55 have a severe mental illness (SMI) and the population of older adults is predicted to double by the year 2030 (U.S. Census Bureau 2000; U.S. Surgeon General 1999a). Patients with SMI include those individuals with schizophrenia, schizoaffective disorders, and bipolar disorders. The needs of this rapidly increasing special population have been overlooked in the public policy debate on how to best organize and finance mental health services. Major public policy issues warranting attention include: 1) converting the system from institution to community-based services, 2) financing of services, 3) integrating mental health and general health care services, and 4) developing innovative models of comprehensive community-based long-term care.

Converting the System from Institutions to Community-Based Services

Until recently, publicly funded services for older adults with SMI have been overwhelmingly provided in institutional settings, including state psychiatric hospitals and nursing homes. Older persons with SMI were the last group to experience the widespread downsizing and closures of long-term inpatient units in the context of deinstitutionalization. Between 1972 and 1987, the number of older state hospital inpatients decreased by 82% (Fogel et al. 1993), followed by additional reductions of 33% between 1986 and 1990 (Atay et al. 1995). However, unlike many younger adults who were discharged to community-based settings, many older persons were "transinstitutionalized" to nursing home beds.

The OBRA '87 nursing home reform legislation regulated and limited the use of nursing homes for the treatment of people with SMI who do not require skilled nursing facility care (Snowden and Roy-Byrne 1998). Despite these regulatory statutes, inappropriate use of nursing home placement of individuals with SMI and other disabilities persists (Office of the Inspector General 2001b). Furthermore, providing nursing home care is cost-intensive and state Medicaid budgets are straining under the burden of supporting institution-based long-term care. In response, supported home- and community-based alternatives to long-term institutional care are receiving considerable attention in meeting the needs and preferences of this population and in limiting the growth of long-term care expenditures (Kane 1998). Of note, despite rapid growth in the population of older persons, the percentage of nursing home residents over age 85 actually declined by 13% between 1985 and 1997 (Health Care Financing Administration 2000c), suggesting that home- and community-based care alternatives have made community residence more likely.

Home- and community-based alternatives are likely to expand as more older adults with SMI reside in these settings (Meeks et al. 1990), especially secondary to Medicaid waivers noted above, and as care providers become more capable of serving chronically ill populations (Institute for Health and Aging 1996). Efforts to find appropriately integrated community-based care have been heightened in recent years due to the 1999 passage of the *Olmstead* decision. This ruling found that placement of disabled individuals in restrictive institutional settings when it is otherwise possible for them to benefit from living in the community constitutes discrimination under the Americans with Disabilities Act (Williams 2000). To comply with the *Olmstead* ruling, states are mandated to develop plans to end unnecessary institutionalization by creating supported opportunities for community living (National Council for Community Behavioral Healthcare 2000). State plans are currently being implemented to review psychiatric inpatients and nursing home residents with disabilities to identify individuals who may benefit from less restrictive settings (National Council for Community Behavioral Healthcare 2000).

Services for Older Adults With Severe Mental Illness: Finance and General Medical Integration

To provide the necessary community-based service infrastructure for older adults with SMI, considerable attention must be focused on efficient and adequate financing of services. Older adults with SMI are among the highest-cost service users. Although they account for the minority (22%) of older adults receiving services in public sector mental health centers, they account for the majority (60%) of mental health service costs. Their treatment is 10 times more expensive than that of persons with depression (Bartels SJ, Miles KM, Dain B, et al.: "Community Mental Health Service Use By Older Adults With Severe Mental Illness," unpublished manuscript, 2002). Over the life cycle, the greatest expenditures per individual with schizophrenia are among the youngest and oldest age groups (Cuffel et al. 1996). Hence, providing appropriate services will require a substantial long-term strategy aimed at identifying the most effective and efficient service models. Despite these costs, current services remain biased toward institutional long-term care with older adults with schizophrenia being substantially at risk for premature and inappropriate nursing home placement (Bartels SJ, Miles KM, Dums AR, et al.: "*Olmstead* and Consumer Vs. Clinician Perspectives on the Most Appropriate Long-Term Setting for Older Adults With Severe Mental Illness," unpublished manuscript, 2002).

Fragmentation of physical and mental health care in primary care and community-based service systems has been a concern for persons with SMI since the beginning of deinstitutionalization. Medical comorbidity is present in nearly all older persons with a significant psychiatric illness (Sheline 1990; Zubenko et al. 1997). Yet despite the high prevalence, medical illnesses among persons served in public sector mental health settings are often undetected by mental health providers (Koran et al. 1989; Koranyi 1979). Medical comorbidity is associated with worse outcomes including greater psychiatric symptoms, morbidity, and mortality (Dalmau et al. 1997; Dixon et al. 1999; Goldman 1999;

Vieweg et al. 1995). Furthermore, older persons with schizophrenia are more likely to die from complications of major medical problems due to inadequate and inappropriate health care (Druss et al. 2001). Ideal models of integrated psychiatric and primary health care include treatment teams with providers that are knowledgeable about the management and interaction of medical and psychiatric illnesses. Public policy addressing future financing and organization of services should prioritize the development and implementation of integrated psychiatric and general health care services for persons with SMI (Mechanic 1997).

To address the issue of cost and fragmentation between mental health and general health care services, many states have implemented managed care arrangements for patients with SMI, including those patients who are older. Most older adults with SMI receive acute and long-term health care services that are financed by FFS Medicare and state Medicaid programs, and in many states Medicaid provides a prescription drug benefit. Ideally, Medicaid carve-in arrangements are well suited for the general older adult population with a variety of psychiatric disorders. However, it has also been argued that carve-out arrangements have the potential to provide higher quality mental health services, especially for older adults with SMI who require specialized services. For example, carve-out organizations employ mental health specialists who are experienced in treating individuals with SMI and are more prepared to provide comprehensive rehabilitative and community support programs for older adults with mental illness (Riley et al. 1997).

Both of these arrangements have inherent problems. Within a carved-in arrangement, mental health services are often a low priority and must compete for funding with other medical specialty services (Bartels et al. 1999). Carved-in mental health care typically offers a limited range of services from providers who are often inadequately trained in mental health and aging. Furthermore, services are often insufficient to meet the intensive care needs of older adults with SMI (Bartels and Colenda 1998; Mechanic 1997). On the other hand, fragmentation of services provided under carved-out arrangements threatens health outcomes for older adults with SMI. Financial incentives may also encourage providers to shift responsibility between medical and mental health providers for addressing comorbid conditions (Bartels et al. 1999). Regardless of the arrangement, Medicare and Medicaid provide the majority of financing of services for older adults with SMI, and projections suggest that the cost of health care will grow exponentially within the next 10 years (Heffler et al. 2002). To meet this growing need, strategies must be developed that are not only cost-effective but also capable of providing appropriate and adequate physical and mental health care.

Innovative Home- and Community-Based Models of Long-Term Care

Several alternatives to traditional financing of long-term care are likely to increase the use and availability of home- and community-based services, including models such as PACE, social HMOs, and long-term care waiver programs. These programs attempt to integrate acute and long-term care services while promoting noninstitutional care settings (Eng et al. 1997; Health Care Financing Administration 2000c; Kane et al. 1997). Medicaid waiver programs offer an alternative to conventional financing and offer flexibility in designating the types of long-term services provided. Recent developments include programs for individuals who are dually eligible for Medicaid and Medicare and multistate proposals that will combine federal Medicaid and Medicare resources in a capitated system (Health Care Financing Administration 2000c). Finally, emerging interventions have the potential to move beyond conventional approaches of providing maintenance long-term care for late-life mental disorders to skills training and cognitive-behavioral therapy (Granholm et al. 2002). Combined with services that provide needed community supports and integrated health care, these models suggest new directions for mental health policy toward improving independent functioning and quality of life for older persons with severe mental illness as they age.

Current Legislative Activity Affecting Geriatric Psychiatry

Although literally hundreds of individual bills addressing health care issues are introduced into the U.S. Congress each year, only a small percentage of those bills are targeted toward the elderly population with mental health concerns. Only about 10% of health care bills introduced into Congress are passed and enacted into law (DeVries and Vanderbilt 1992). It is rare that a fully developed legislative proposal enacting any type of sweeping change is adopted by Congress in a short period of time (less than 5 years). The path of legislation from introduction of a bill to final passage is intentionally filled with many challenges and pitfalls as a means to ensure that a final law has been thoroughly discussed prior to enactment.

Numerous bills are pending in Congress that would have some impact on the access to quality mental health services under today's health care delivery system, including coverage of prescription drugs, Medicare reform, mental health parity, and long-term care reform.

Mental Health Parity

Approximately 98% of private health insurance plans discriminate against patients seeking treatment for mental illness by requiring higher copayments or higher deductibles or by allowing fewer doctor visits or days in the hospital than for other medical illnesses (American Association for Geriatric Psychiatry 2001). A key component of any mental health advocacy agenda is the realization of parity for mental health services with those of other medical services. Health care consumers requiring treatment for mental illness continue to be discriminated against as they receive lower copayments, limitations on reimbursement, and other arbitrary restrictions. A variety of approaches to achieving mental health parity have been utilized by both federal and state legislative bodies; these range from narrowly defined proposals mandating that lifetime limits on health insurance be equal for medical and mental illness benefits to very broad proposals that significantly overhaul the payment system for mental health insurance benefits. For example, a federal law that prohibits a lesser amount of lifetime limits to benefits for mental health services has been in effect for several years. In addition, by federal executive order, federal employees began receiving parity benefits in their health plans in January 2001. However, disparity in reimbursement is still prevalent. Most recently, legislation has been introduced and considered by Congress that would ensure greater parity in the coverage of mental health benefits by prohibiting a group health plan from treating mental health benefits differently from the coverage of medical and surgical benefits. Specifically, group health plans would not be able to set different limits or financial requirements in such areas as patient copayments and deductibles, length of hospital stays, and number of outpatient visits. This legislation was passed by the Senate in 2001 but has not achieved final passage.

Although the adoption of mental health parity legislation appears to be noncontroversial, there are several areas of dispute by lawmakers. For example, coverage of alcohol and drug abuse as a mental illness has been a long-fought issue in both houses of Congress. Other legislators argue that mandating mental health parity is cost prohibitive to small businesses. Most of the mental health parity proposals would exempt companies with fewer than 50 employees from the mandate.

Mental health parity under Medicare continues to receive some legislative attention. During a recent session of Congress, legislation was introduced to end the historic discrimination against Medicare beneficiaries seeking outpatient treatment for mental illness as well as eliminate the 190-day lifetime cap on inpatient services in psychiatric hospitals. To date, no action has been taken by Congress.

Federal Training Funds

Geriatric psychiatry is a relatively small medical specialty, but it is one for which demand is increasing rapidly as the population ages. The ability to provide access to quality mental health services for the elderly in the future will be directly affected by the pipeline of medical education programs that produce physicians specializing in geriatric care.

Legislation has been introduced that would increase the number of physicians specializing in geriatric care through training incentives and greater Medicare reimbursement. Under the BBA-97, the total number of full-time equivalent (FTE) interns and residents for which Medicare would pay the direct costs of medical education was capped at each teaching hospital. A facility's cap is based on the number of FTEs it had in 1996. Since the cap is applied in the aggregate, a teaching hospital may increase the number of FTEs in one specialty if it makes offsetting reductions in the number FTEs in other specialties. This cap also limits the number of FTEs that are counted in determining a hospital's Medicare payment adjustment for the indirect costs of medical education. Under current law, hospitals receive 100% GME reimbursement for an individual's initial residency period up to 5 years. The law also includes a geriatric exception allowing programs training geriatric fellows to receive full funding for an additional period composed of the first and second years of fellowship training. Programs training nongeriatric fellows receive 50% of GME funding for fellowship training. In 1998, the period of board eligibility for geriatrics was decreased to 1 year in an effort to encourage more geriatric specialists.

Congress is considering a proposal to add up to five FTEs in geriatric residency or fellowship programs (above the 1996 levels) without reducing the number of FTEs in other specialties. Geriatric residency or fellowship programs include programs in medicine or psychiatry. The legislation would explicitly authorize full Medicare GME payments for the second year of fellowship.

Seclusion and Restraint Regulations

There has been a general public outcry about the inappropriate use of seclusion and restraint for patients of hospitals and nursing homes, including the use of chemical restraints. Seclusion and restraints are medical interventions that are sometimes required for some psychiatry patients (e.g., to prevent harm to the patient or to ensure a safe treatment environment); however, the regulations governing use of these methods are contradictory and confusing. Since 1999, different regulatory bodies have issued four separate overlapping national standards on the appropriate use of seclusion and restraints. CMS is currently attempting to write one standard set of guidelines for the use of chemical restraints. In January 2001, CMS issued draft language for nursing home surveyor guidelines for review of chemical restraints. The CMS received literally thousands of responses to that draft language and subsequently convened a task force to put further work into the development of the guidelines. In May 2001, the OIG issued a report stating that there was little or no evidence that psychotropic drugs were being used inappropriately as chemical restraints in nursing homes. Although some advocates thought that the OIG report would terminate any additional CMS activity on chemical restraints, a final proposal on appropriate chemical restraint use is expected in 2002.

Privacy and Confidentiality

The Health Insurance Portability and Accountability Act of 1996 (HIPAA) included provisions designed to lower costs for the health care industry by requiring adoption of federal transaction standards for electronic transfers of health care information. At the same time, HIPPA required the adoption of new safeguards to protect the security and confidentiality of that information. The final regulations governing privacy and confidentiality of patient records were issued in December 2000 and took effect in April 2001. The rule covers all individually identifiable health information used or disclosed by a covered entity in any form. It provides new rights for patients to understand and control how their health information is used; generally limits use of an individual's health information to health purposes; establishes the privacy safeguard standards that covered entities must meet; and establishes accountability for medical records and release. These new rules affect both geriatric psychiatry practices as well as the use of patient data for research purposes, although the final rule contains special provisions for psychotherapy notes.

Summary

Late-life mental disorders are prevalent illnesses that have a significant impact on the quality of life for older adults. Treatment for these disorders is inextricably linked to primary care, and for frail elderly patients, clinicians must consider how medical-psychiatric comorbidity affects treatment decisions and outcomes. The system of care—how it is structured, financed, and regulated—is in considerable flux. Financing is typically less generous than for other medical conditions, and the government plays the largest role in underwriting expenditures for the elderly. Additionally, contradictory federal regulatory policy that requires mental health assessment and treatment in long-term care settings collides with both practice and payment policy.

Even while the BBA-97 attempts to incentivize older adults to enroll in Medicare managed care programs, managed care plans are dropping out of Medicare, resulting in slower growth over the past 2 years. Similarly, state Medicaid managed care initiatives are creating opportunities to reallocate support to the development of home- and community-based alternative models of care, with the goal of supporting least-restrictive and less-costly long-term care services for the elderly. Substantial concern exists, however, that those who have the highest requirements for comprehensive wrap-around services will go wanting. Yet to be determined is the impact of these types of programs on overall health and well-being, improved quality of life, and access to needed mental health services. Recent federal legislative initiatives focusing on Medicare parity and reform, seclusion and restraint, and patient privacy have not come to grips with the central overriding fact that by 2020, perhaps as many as 9 million elderly will have a clinically significant mental disorder. Thus, driven by current economic and cost containment forces, the configuration of and the long-term outcomes for mental health services to the elderly remain unclear.

References

American Association for Geriatric Psychiatry: Legislative and Regulatory Agenda, 2001–2002. Bethesda, MD, American Association for Geriatric Psychiatry, 2001

American Association of Health Plans: Facts in Brief: Enrollment Demographics in Medicare HMOs. Washington, DC, American Association of Health Plans, 2000

Atay JE, Witkin MJ, Manderscheid RW: Data Highlights On Utilization of Mental Health Organizations by Elderly Persons [DHHS Publ. No. SMA 95-3032]. Washington, DC, U.S. Government Printing Office, 1995

Avorn J, Soumerai SD, Everitt DE, et al: A randomized trial of a program to reduce the use of psychoactive drugs in nursing homes. N Engl J Med 327:168–173, 1992

Bartels SJ, Colenda CC: Mental health services for Alzheimer's disease: current trends in reimbursement and public policy, and the future under managed care. Am J Geriatr Psychiatry 6:S85–S100, 1998

Bartels SJ, Levine KJ, Shea D: Community-based long-term care for older persons with severe and persistent mental illness in an era of managed care. Psychiatr Serv 50:1189–1197, 1999

Borson S, Loebel JP, Kitchell M, et al: Psychiatric assessments of nursing home residents under OBRA-87: should PASARR be reformed? Preadmission screening and annual review. J Am Geriatr Soc 45:1173–1181, 1997

Borson S, Bartels SJ, Colenda CC, et al: Geriatric mental health services research: strategic plan for an aging population. Report of the health services work group of the American Association for Geriatric Psychiatry. Am J Geriatr Psychiatry 9:191–204, 2001

Cano C, Hennessy K, Warren J, et al: Medicare Part A utilization and expenditures for psychiatric services: 1995. Health Care Financ Rev 18:177–194, 1997

Centers for Medicare and Medicaid Services: National Health Expenditures: 2000–2010. Washington DC, U.S. Government Printing Office, 2001. Available online at http://www.hcfa.gov/stats/nhe-oact/hilites.htm. Accessed February 2002.

Centers for Medicare and Medicaid Services: Your Medicare Benefits. Washington DC, U.S. Government Printing Office, 2002. Available online at http://www.medicare.gov/Publications/Pubs/pdf/10116.pdf. Accessed February 22, 2003.

Centers for Medicare and Medicaid Services: Medicare Managed Care Contract (MMCC) Plans: Monthly Summary Report. Washington, DC, U.S. Government Printing Office, January 2003. Available online at http://cms.hhs.gov/healthplans/statistics/MMCC. Accessed February 22, 2003.

Colenda CC, Streim JE, Greene JA, et al: The impact of the Omnibus Budget Reconciliation Act of 1987 (OBRA'87) on psychiatric services in nursing homes. Am J Geriatr Psychiatry 7:12–17, 1999

Colenda CC, Bartels SC, Gottlieb GL: The North American system of care, in Principles and Practice of Geriatric Psychiatry, 2nd Edition. Edited by Copeland J, Abou-Saleh M, Blazer D. London, England, John Wiley & Sons, 2002, pp 689–696

Cuffel BJ, Jeste DV, Halpain M, et al: Treatment costs and use of community mental health services for schizophrenia by age cohorts. Am J Psychiatry 153:870–876, 1996

Dalmau A, Bergman B, BrismarB: Somatic morbidity in schizophrenia: a case control study. Public Health 111:393–397, 1997

DeVries C, Vanderbilt M: The Grassroots Lobbying Handbook. Washington, DC, American Nurses Association, 1992

Dixon L, Postrado L, Delahanty J, et al: The association of medical comorbidity in schizophrenia with poor physical and mental health. J Nerv Ment Dis 187:496–502, 1999

Druss BG, Bradford WD, Rosenheck RA, et al: Quality of medical care and excess mortality in older patients with mental disorders. Arch Gen Psychiatry 58:565–572, 2001

Eng C, Pedulla J, Eleazer GP, et al: Program of all-inclusive care for the elderly (PACE): an innovative model of integrated geriatric care and financing. J Am Geriatr Soc 45:223–232, 1997

Fogel BS: The United States' system of care, in Principles and Practices of Geriatric Psychiatry. Edited by Copeland JRM, Abou-Saleh MT, Blazer DG. London, England, John Wiley & Sons, 1994, pp 923–931

Fogel BS, Colenda CC, Moak G, et al: Geriatric Psychiatry in State Hospitals: Task Force Report on Public Psychiatry and Geriatrics. Washington, DC, American Psychiatric Association, 1993

Frank RG: The creation of Medicare and Medicaid: the emergence of insurance and markets for mental health services. Psychiatr Serv 51:465–468, 2000

Frank RG, McGuire TG, Bae JP, et al: Solutions for adverse selection in behavioral healthcare. Health Care Financ Rev 18:109–122, 1997

Goldman LS: Medical illness in patients with schizophrenia. J Clin Psychiatry 60(suppl 21):10–15, 1999

Granholm E, McQuaid JR, McClure FS, et al: A randomized controlled pilot study of cognitive behavioral social skills training for older patients with schizophrenia. Schizophr Res 53:167–169, 2002

Health Care Financing Administration: Medicare and Medicaid: requirements for long-term care facilities, final regulations. Federal Register 56:48865–48921, 1991

Health Care Financing Administration: Medicare and Medicaid Programs: preadmission screening and annual resident review. Federal Register 57:56450–56504, 1992a

Health Care Financing Administration: Medicare and Medicaid: resident assessment in long-term care facilities. Federal Register 57:61614–61733, 1992b

Health Care Financing Administration: Medicare 2000: 35 years of Improving Americans' Health and Security. Washington DC, U.S. Government Printing Office, 2000a. Available online at http://cms.hhs.gov/statistics/35chartbk.pdf. Accessed February 22, 2003.

Health Care Financing Administration: Medicare and Your Mental Health Benefits. Washington DC, U.S. Government Printing Office, 2000b

Health Care Financing Administration: A Profile of Medicaid: Chartbook 2000. Washington, DC, Department of Health and Human Services, 2000c

Heffler S, Smith S, Won G, et al: Health spending projections for 2001–2011: the latest outlook. Health Affairs 21:207–218, 2002

Institute for Health and Aging: Chronic Care in America: A 21st Century Challenge. Princeton, NJ, Robert Wood Johnson Foundation, 1996

Institute of Medicine, Committee on Improving Quality in Long-Term Care: Improving the Quality of Long-Term Care. Edited by Wunderlich GS, Kohler P. Washington DC, National Academy Press, 2001

Institute of Medicine, Committee on Nursing Home Regulation: Improving the Quality of Care in Nursing Homes. Washington DC, National Academy Press, 1986

Kane RL: Managed care as a vehicle for delivering more effective chronic care for older persons. J Am Geriatr Soc 46:1034–1039, 1998

Kane RL, Kane RA, Finch M, et al: S/HMOs, the second generation: building on the experience of the first social health maintenance organization demonstrations. J Am Geriatr Soc 45:101–107, 1997

Koran LM, Sox HC, Marton KL, et al: Medical evaluation of psychiatric patients. Arch Gen Psychiatry 46:733–740, 1989

Koranyi EK: Morbidity and rate of undiagnosed physical illnesses in a psychiatric clinic population. Arch Gen Psychiatry 36:14–19, 1979

Langwell K, Topoleski C, Sherman D: Analysis of Benefits Offered by Medicare HMOs, 1999: Complexities and Implications. Menlo Park, CA, Henry J. Kaiser Foundation, 1999

Levit K, Smith C, Cowan C, et al: Inflation spurs health spending in 2000. Health Affairs 21:172–181, 2002

Llorente MD, Olsen EJ, Leyva O, et al: Use of antipsychotic drugs in nursing homes: current compliance with OBRA regulations. J Am Geriatr Soc 46:198–201, 1998

Marino S, Gallo D, Anthony JC: Filters on the pathway to mental health care, I: incident mental disorders. Psychol Med 25:1135–1148, 1995

Mark T, McKusick D, King E, et al: National Expenditures for Mental Health, Alcohol, and other Drug Abuse Treatment, 1996. Substance Abuse and Mental Health Services Administration. Washington DC, U.S. Government Printing Office, 1998

Mechanic D: Approaches for coordinating primary and specialty care for persons with mental illness. Gen Hosp Psychiatry 19:395–402, 1997

Medicare Payment Advisory Commission: Beneficiaries' financial liability and Medicare's effectiveness in reducing personal spending, in Medicare Payment Advisory Commission Report to Congress: Selected Medicare Issues. Washington, DC, Medicare Payment Advisory Commission, 1999a, pp 3–15

Medicare Payment Advisory Commission: A framework for considering Medicare payment policy issues, in Medicare Payment Advisory Commission Report to Congress: Medicare Payment Policy. Washington, DC, Medicare Payment Advisory Commission, 1999b, pp 3–24

Medicare Payment Advisory Commission: Medicare + choice: a program in transition, in Medicare Payment Advisory Commission Report to Congress: Medicare Payment Policy. Washington DC, Medicare Payment Advisory Commission, 1999c, pp 27–46

Medicare Program: Medicare + Choice Fact Sheet. Menlo Park, CA, Henry J. Kaiser Family Foundation, June 2002. Available online at http://www.kff.org/content/2002/2052-04/2052-04.pdf. Accessed February 22, 2003.

Meeks S, Carstensen LL, Stafford PB, et al: Mental health needs of the chronically mentally ill elderly. Psychol Aging 5:163–171, 1990

Mickus M, Colenda CC, Hogan AJ: Knowledge of mental health benefits and preferences for type of mental health providers among the general public. Psychiatr Serv 51:199–202, 2002

Mollica RL, Riley T: Managed Care, Medicaid and the Elderly: An Overview of Five State Case Studies. Minneapolis, MN, University of Minnesota National Long Term Care Resource Center, 1996

Narrow WE, Rae DS, Robins LN, et al: Revised prevalence estimates of mental disorders in the United States. Arch Gen Psychiatry 59:115–123, 2002

National Council for Community Behavioral Healthcare: Olmstead: Department of Health and Human Services Urges Implementation of Olmstead. Rockville, MD, National Council for Community Behavioral Healthcare, 2000. Available online at http://www.nccbh.org/html/policy/archives/olmstead.htm. Accessed February 22, 2003.

Office of the Inspector General: Mental Health Services in Nursing Facilities (OEI-02–91–00860). Washington, DC, U.S. Department of Health and Human Services, 1996

Office of the Inspector General: Medicare Part B Payments for Mental Health Services (OEI-03–99–00130). Department of Health and Human Services. Washington DC, U.S. Government Printing Office, 2001a

Office of the Inspector General: Medicare Payments for Psychiatric Services in Nursing Homes: A Follow-up (OEI-02–99–00140). Washington, DC, U.S. Department of Health and Human Services, 2001b

Omnibus Budget Reconciliation Act of 1987 [P.L. 100–203]. Washington, DC, U.S. Government Printing Office, 1987. Available online at http://thomas.loc.gov/cgi-bin/bdquery/z?d100:HR03545: | TOM:/bss/d100query.html |. Accessed February 22, 2003.

Physician Payment Review Commission: Medicaid: spending trends and the move to managed care, in Physician Payment Review Commission: Annual Report to Congress, 1997. Washington, DC, Physician Payment Review Commission, 1997, pp 412–448

Regier DA, Meyers JK, Kramer M, et al: The NIMH Epidemiologic Catchment Area program: historical context, major objectives, and population characteristics. Arch Gen Psychiatry 41:934–941, 1984

Regier DA, Narrow WE, Rae DS, et al: The de facto U.S. metal and addictive disorders service system: Epidemiologic Catchment Area prospective 1-year prevalence rates of disorders and services. Arch Gen Psychiatry 50:85–94, 1993

Riley T, Rawlings-Sekunda J, Pernice C: Medicaid managed care and mental health, in Medicaid Managed Care: A Guide for States, 3rd Edition, Vol 4: Challenges and Solutions: Medicaid Managed Care Programs Serving the Elderly and Persons with Disabilities. Portland, ME, National Academy for State Health Policy, 1997, pp 79–101

Rovner BW, Edelman BA, Cox MP, et al: The impact of antipsychotic drug regulations (OBRA 1987) on psychotropic prescribing practices in nursing homes. Am J Psychiatry 149:1390–1392, 1992

Semla TP, Palla K, Poddig B, et al: Effect of the Omnibus Reconciliation Act 1987 on antipsychotic prescribing in nursing home residents. J Am Geriatr Soc 42:648–652, 1994

Shea D: Economic and financial issues in mental health and aging. The Public Policy and Aging Report 9:7–12, 1998

Sheline YI: High prevalence of physical illness in a geriatric psychiatric inpatient population. Gen Hosp Psychiatry 12:396–400, 1990

Sherman J: Medicare's Mental Health Benefits: Coverage Utilization and Expenditures, 1992. Washington, DC, American Association of Retired Persons, Public Policy Institute, 1992

Shorr RI, Fought RL, Ray WA: Changes in antipsychotic drug use in nursing homes during implementation of the OBRA-87 regulations. JAMA 271:358–362, 1994

Siegler EL, Capezuti E, Maislin G, et al: Effects of a restraint reduction intervention and OBRA '87 regulations on psychoactive drug use in nursing homes. J Am Geriatr Soc 45:791–796, 1997

Snowden M, Roy-Byrne P: Mental illness and nursing home reform: OBRA-87 ten years later. Omnibus Budget Reconciliation Act. Psychiatr Serv 49:229–233, 1998

Streim JE, Beckwith EW, Arapakos D, et al: Payment Policy, Regulatory Oversight, and Quality Improvement in the Provision of Mental Health Services in Nursing Homes. Psychiatr Serv 53:1414–1418, 2002

U.S. Census Bureau: 65+ in the United States, P23–190. Current Population Reports, Special Studies. Washington, DC, U.S. Government Printing Office, 1996, Table 2–1

U.S. Census Bureau: Projections of the Resident Population by Age, Sex, Race, and Hispanic Origin: 1999–2100. Population Projections Program, Population Division. Washington, DC, U.S. Department of Commerce, 2000

U.S. Census Bureau: Profiles of General Demographic Characteristics: 2000 Census of Population and Housing, United States. Washington, DC, U.S. Department of Commerce, 2001

U.S. Surgeon General: Older adults and mental health, in Mental Health: A Report of the Surgeon General. Rockville, MD, Department of Health and Human Services, 1999a, pp 335–401

U.S. Surgeon General: Organizing and financing mental health services, in Mental Health: A Report of the Surgeon General. Rockville, MD, Department of Health and Human Services, 1999b, pp 405–433

U.S. Surgeon General: Mental Health: A Report of the Surgeon General. Rockville, MD, Department of Health and Human Services, 1999c

Vieweg V, Levenson J, Pandurangi A, et al: Medical disorders in the schizophrenic patient. Int J Psychiatry Med 25:137–172, 1995

Wells KB, Astrachan BM, Tischler GL, et al: Issues and approaches in evaluating managed mental health care. Milbank Q 73:57–75, 1995

Williams L: Long-term care after Olmstead v. L.C.: will the potential of the ADA's integration mandate be achieved? J Contemp Health Law Policy 17:205–239, 2000

Witkin MJ, Atay JE, Manderscheid RW, et al: Highlights of organized mental health services in 1994 and major national and state trends, in Mental Health United States, 1998 [Publ. No. (SMA) 99–3285]. Edited by Manderscheid RW, Henderson MJ. Washington, DC, Department of Health and Human Services, 1998, pp 143–175

Zubenko GS, Marino LJ, Sweet RA, et al: Medical comorbidity in elderly psychiatric inpatients. Biol Psychiatry 41:724–736, 1997

Index

*Page numbers printed in **boldface** type refer to tables or figures.*

Aphasias, and frontotemporal dementias, 41. *See also* Language

Apolipoprotein E (ApoE), and Alzheimer's disease, 46–47

Aspirin, and vascular dementia, 61, 62

Assessment. *See also* Diagnosis
of alcohol abuse, 114–116
of depression in dementia, 6

Atypical antipsychotics. *See also* Antipsychotics
bipolar disorder and, 87
delusional disorder and, 89
dementia with Lewy bodies and, 41
frontotemporal dementias and, 95
medication-induced psychosis and, 100
psychotic symptoms due to medical illness and, 97
side effects of, 102

Balanced Budget Act of 1997, 151

Barbiturates, and alcohol interactions, **120**

Behavior. *See also* Aggression; Disinhibition
frontotemporal dementias and disturbances in, 95
psychotic symptoms in dementia and, 91–92
treatment for symptoms of Alzheimer's disease, 55, 58–60

Behavioral interventions. *See also* Cognitive behavioral therapy
for alcohol abuse, 122
for depression in dementia, 14

Beliefs, and dementias, 90

Benign organic hallucinosis, 98

Benzodiazepines
alcohol detoxification and, 126
alcohol interactions and, **119**
anxiety disorders and, 21
delirium and, 96
psychotic symptoms and abuse of, 102
treatment for abuse of, 130–131
withdrawal from abuse of, 130

Berlin Aging Study (BASE), 15

Beta amyloid, and Alzheimer's disease, 44, 57

Binge drinking, and treatment outcome, 129

Bipolar disorder
cardiovascular and pulmonary mortality in, 79, 86
prevalence of in elderly, 76
psychoses associated with, 86–87

Brief interventions, and alcohol abuse, 121–123

Brief psychotic disorder, 89

Buffalo Creek Dam collapse, 18

Bupropion, and depression, 3

Buspirone, and anxiety disorders, 21

CAGE, 115

Capgras' syndrome, 91

Carbamazepine, and anxiety disorders, 21

Caregivers, of Alzheimer's disease patients, 44, 58, 59, 60, 64–65

Carve-out and carve-in plans, for mental health care, 154–155, 166–167

Catatonia, and bipolar disorder, 86

Centers for Medicare and
Medicaid Services (CMS),
147, 162–163, 171
Center for Substance Abuse
Treatment (CSAT), and
Treatment Improvement
Protocol (TIP), 113–114
Cerebrovascular disease. *See also*
Stroke
bipolar disorder and, 79, 86
vascular dementia and, 94
Cholesterol levels, and
Alzheimer's disease, 47
Cholinesterase inhibitors. *See also*
Donazepil; Tacrine
Alzheimer's disease and, 38,
51–55, 93
contraindications for, 54
dementia with Lewy bodies
and, 41, 95
depression in dementia and,
13
psychotic symptoms in
dementia and, 92
Chromosome 17-linked multiple
system tauopathy, 43
Chronic mental illness,
prevalence of in elderly, 76
Chronic obstructive pulmonary
disease (COPD), and anxiety
disorders, 21
Cimetidine, and medication-
induced psychotic
symptoms, **101**
Citalopram, and psychotic
symptoms in dementia, 92
Clomipramine
anxiety disorders and, 21
depression in dementia and, **10**
Clopidogrel, and vascular
dementia, 61

Clozapine
bipolar disorder and, 87
dosing in elderly, **103**
psychosis in context of
epilepsy and, 98
psychotic symptoms in
Parkinson's disease and, 99
schizophrenia and, 84–85
side effects in older patients,
102
Cognitive behavioral therapy
(CBT), and anxiety disorders,
21–22. *See also* Behavioral
interventions
Cognitive enrichment programs, 65
Cognitive impairment. *See also*
Cognitive rehabilitation;
Memory
alcohol abuse and, 120–121
clinical expression of
depression in dementia
and, 4
diagnosis of depression in
elderly and, 2
Lewy body disease and, 94
pseudodementia and, 7
psychoses associated with Alzheimer's disease and, 93
Cognitive rehabilitation. *See also*
Cognitive impairment;
Rehabilitation
Alzheimer's disease and,
64–65
traumatic brain injury and,
63–64
vascular dementia and, 62
Combat veterans, and
posttraumatic stress disorder,
17, 18–19
Comfort zone, for Alzheimer's
patients, 59

Community-based services
  models of long-term care and,
    167
  severe mental illness and,
    163–164
Community-based studies, of
  late-life depression, 1–2
Comorbidity
  alcohol abuse and, 131–136
  of depression with medical
    illness, 2
  of generalized anxiety disorder
    with medical illness, 19
  obsessive-compulsive
    disorder and, 18–19
  of panic disorder with medical
    illness, 16
  psychotic disorders and, 77,
    78–79
Compliance, with treatment
  for delusional disorder, 89
  for substance abuse, 126–128
Confidentiality, in geriatric
  psychiatry, 171
Cornell Scale for Depression in
  Dementia (CSDD), 8–9
Cortisol levels, and depression in
  dementia, 5–6
Creutzfeldt-Jakob disease, 36
Crime, and phobias, 20
Cultural stigma, of mental illness,
  151

Death, suicide and leading causes
  of, 135. *See also* Mortality rates
Deinstitutionalization, and
  severe mental illness, 163
Delirium
  Parkinson's disease and, 99
  psychotic symptoms
    associated with, 95–96

Delusional depression, 88
Delusional disorder, 88–89
Delusional parasitosis, 89
Delusions
  dementia and, 90
  delirium and, 96
  frontotemporal dementias
    and, 95
  medical illness and, 97
  psychoses associated with Alz-
    heimer's disease and, 93
  schizophrenia and, 82, 83
  vascular dementia and, 94
Dementia
  alcoholism and, 136
  Alzheimer's disease and,
    43–60
  depression and, 3–14
  diagnosis of, 35–36
  health care expenditures and,
    149
  psychotic symptoms and,
    90–92
  PTSD symptoms and, 18
  schizophrenia and, 78
  types of, 38–66
Dementia of the Alzheimer's
  type, and psychotic
  symptoms, 81, 91
Dementia Mood Assessment
  Scale (DMAS), 8
Dementia with Lewy bodies (DLB)
  cholinesterase inhibitors and, 55
  diagnosis of, 40–41
  pathophysiology of, 38–40, 47
  prevalence of depression in, 5
  psychotic symptoms and, 91
  treatment of, 41, 94–95
Department of Health and
  Human Services, 149–150,
  161–163

Estrogen, and Alzheimer's disease, 56
Extrapyramidal symptoms (EPS), and antipsychotics, 77, 84, 103

Falls, and dementia with Lewy bodies, 40
Family history, of psychotic symptoms, 79
Fluoxetine
  anxiety disorders and, 21
  comorbid alcoholism and depression, 133–134
Fluvoxamine, and anxiety disorders, 20
Folic acid, and Alzheimer's disease, 48, 62
Frontotemporal dementias (FTDs)
  Alzheimer's disease, Lewy body variant of AD, and diffuse Lewy body disease compared to, **45**
  associated conditions, 42–43
  clinical presentations of, 41
  diagnosis of, 41–42
  psychosis associated with, 95
  treatment of, 43
Full-time equivalent (FTE) interns and residents, 170

Gabapentin, and anxiety disorders, 21
Galantamine, and Alzheimer's disease, 52, 54
Generalized anxiety disorder
  epidemiology of, 19
  prevalence of in elderly, 15
Government. *See* Public policy; States

Gross domestic product, and national health expenditures, 147
Guy's/Age Concern Survey, 15

Hallucinations
  Alzheimer's disease and, 58, 93
  delirium and, 96
  delusional disorder and, 89
  dementia with Lewy bodies and, 40
  Lewy body disease and, 94
  ophthalmological disorders and, 99–100
  Parkinson's disease and, 98, 99
  psychotic symptoms and, 90–91
  schizophrenia and, 82, 83
  vascular dementia and, 94
Haloperidol
  delirium and, 96
  dementia with Lewy bodies and, 95
Hamilton Rating Scale for Depression (HRSD), 8
Head injury, as risk factor for Alzheimer's disease, 46–47. *See also* Traumatic brain injury
Health care. *See also* Medical conditions; Public policy
  alcohol use and, 111, 114
  increasing need and demand for by older adults, 111, 112
  primary care providers and depression in elderly, 2–3
  services utilization by patients with depression in dementia, 9
  severe mental illness and medical integration, 165–167

Health Care Financing Administration (HCFA), 159, 160, 161, 162

Health insurance, and mental health parity, 168–169. *See also* Medicaid; Medicare

Health Insurance Portability and Accountability Act of 1996 (HIPAA), 171

Health maintenance organizations (HMOs), and Medicare, 152–153, 167

Herbal remedies, and polypharmacy, 104

Hoarding, and obsessive-compulsive disorder, 17

Holocaust survivors, and post-traumatic stress disorder, 18

Home-based model, for long-term care, 167

Homocysteine levels, and Alzheimer's disease, 47–48

Hydroxychloroquine, and Alzheimer's disease, 57

Hypercholesterolemia, and Alzheimer's disease, 47

Hypercortisolemia, and depression in dementia, 5–6

Hyperhomocysteinemia
Alzheimer's disease and, 47–48
vascular dementia and, 62

Hypolipidemic agents, and vascular dementia, 62

Imipramine
anxiety disorders and, 20
comorbid alcoholism and depression, 133
depression in dementia and, **10**

Incontinence, and Alzheimer's disease, 60

Indomethacin, and cognitive function, 56

Infectious diseases, and psychotic symptoms, **97**

Inpatient mental health care, and Medicare, 152

Institute of Medicine (IOM), 158–159, 160–161

Intellectual activity, and Alzheimer's disease, 48–51

Interpersonal interventions, for depression in dementia, 14

Korean War, and posttraumatic stress disorder in veterans, 18–19

Laboratory tests, and psychotic symptoms due to medical illness, 97

Language. *See also* Aphasias
frontotemporal dementias and impairment of, 95
schizophrenia and production of, 83

Late onset schizophrenia (LOS), 82–85

Legislation, and geriatric psychiatry, 168–171

Lewy bodies, diseases associated with, 39

Lewy body variant of AD (LBV)
Alzheimer's disease, diffuse Lewy body disease, and frontotemporal dementias compared to, **45**
diagnosis of, 40–41
pathophysiology of, 39–40
psychoses associated with, 94–95

Lifestyle, and alcohol use, 111

Lithium
　　Alzheimer's disease and, 58
　　bipolar disorder and, 87
Living arrangements, and
　　treatment of substance abuse,
　　126
Locus caeruleus, and
　　Alzheimer's disease, 5
Longitudinal Aging Study of
　　Amsterdam (LASA), 15
Long-term care
　　home- and community-based
　　　models of, 167
　　Medicaid and, 156–163

Managed care plans
　　Medicare and, 151, 152–153
　　severe mental illness and,
　　　166
Mania
　　bipolar disorder and, 86
　　new onset of in later life, 81
　　overlap of with delirium, 96
Medicaid, and financing of long-
　　term care, 156–163, 166, 167
Medical conditions. *See also*
　　Health care
　　alcohol abuse and comorbidity
　　　with, 131–136
　　depression and comorbidity
　　　with, 2
　　generalized anxiety disorder
　　　and comorbidity with, 19
　　panic disorder and
　　　comorbidity with, 16
　　psychoses due to, 96–98
　　psychotic disorders and
　　　comorbidity with, 77, 78
　　severe mental illness and
　　　comorbidity with,
　　　165–166

Medicare. *See also* Public policy
　　mental health expenditures
　　　and, 149–151
　　parity for mental health care,
　　　155
　　reform of, 156
　　severe mental illness and, 166
　　trends in health expenditures
　　　and, 148
Medicare Risk Contracting
　　(MRC) Plans, 152, 154
Medication-induced psychosis,
　　98–99, 100, **101**
Medications, and potential
　　interaction with alcohol, 113.
　　See also Prescription drugs;
　　Psychoactive medications
Memory, Alzheimer's disease
　　and deficits in, 36–37, 38, 65.
　　See also Cognitive impairment
Mental activity, and Alzheimer's
　　disease, 48–51
Metabolic disorders, and
　　psychotic symptoms, **97**
Mild cognitive impairment, and
　　Alzheimer's disease, 36–38
Mini-Mental State Examination,
　　49, 52
Mirtazapine, and depression, 3
Moclobemide, and depression in
　　dementia, **10**
Mood disturbances, and
　　Alzheimer's disease, 58
Mood stabilizers, and bipolar
　　disorder, 87
Mortality rates, and bipolar
　　disorder, 79, 86. *See also* Death

Naltrexone, and alcoholism, 126,
　　134
Narcotics Anonymous, 125

Opiate/opioid analgesics, and
alcohol interactions, **119–120**.
See also Analgesics
Outcome research, on substance
abuse, 129–130
Outpatient services,
underutilization of, 150
Over-the-counter medications,
and psychotic symptoms, **101**

Panic disorder, 15–16
Parkinson's disease (PD)
Lewy bodies and, 39
psychotic symptoms and,
98–99
Pathophysiology
of dementia with Lewy bodies,
38–41, 47
of depression in dementia, 5–6
of schizophrenia, 82–83
of vascular dementia, 60
Phenothiazines, and alcohol
interactions, **120**
Phobias and phobic disorders, 15,
19–20
Pick's disease, 41–42
Point of Service (POS) Options,
152–153
Polypharmacy, and adverse
reactions, 103–104
Posttraumatic stress disorder
(PTSD)
epidemiology of, 17–19
hallucinations and differential
diagnosis of, 90
Preadmission screening and
annual resident review
(PASARR), 159, 160
Predementia, 7
Prednisone, and Alzheimer's
disease, 56–57

Prescription drugs. *See also*
Psychoactive medications
abuse of, 113
alcohol use and interactions
with, 116, 131
psychosis induced by, 100, **101**
Prevalence. *See also*
Epidemiology
of alcohol abuse, 112–113, 136
of anxiety disorders, 14–15
of depression in Alzheimer's
disease, 5, 8
of depression in dementia, 4–5
of generalized anxiety
disorder, 19
of late-life depression, 1–2
of mental illness in older
adults, 145–146, 150
of obsessive-compulsive
disorder, 15, 16
of panic disorder, 15–16
of phobias, 20
of posttraumatic stress
disorder, 18
of psychotic disorders, 75–76
of vascular dementia, 94
Prevention, of vascular dementia,
62
Primary progressive aphasia
(PPA), 41
Primary psychotic disorders, 77,
78, 82–90
Prisoners-of-war (POWs),
and posttraumatic
stress disorder, 18
Privacy, and rules affecting
geriatric psychiatry, 171
Prodromal symptoms, and
depression in dementia, 4
Programs of All-Inclusive Care for
the Elderly (PACE), 152, 167

Sleep-wake disturbances and
  sleep disorders
  alcohol use and, 136
  Alzheimer's disease and, 60
  Parkinson's disease and, 99
Social Darwinism, and health
  care policy, 146
Social isolation, and psychosis in
  elderly, 76
Social phobia, 20
Social roles, and alcohol use, 121
Social Security Act of 1965, 156, 158
Social services
  nursing homes and, 161
  substance abuse and, 126
Sodium valproate, and anxiety
  disorders, 21
States, and Medicaid financing of
  long-term care, 156–163
Statin drugs
  Alzheimer's disease and, 47, 48
  vascular dementia and, 62
Steroids, and medication-induced
  psychotic symptoms, **101**
Stimulants, and medication-
  induced psychotic
  symptoms, **101**
Stroke. *See also* Cerebrovascular
  disease
  alcohol abuse and, 131
  apathy and depression in, 6
  vascular dementia and, 61
Substance use disorders. *See also*
  Alcoholism and alcohol abuse
  assessment of, 115
  depression and, 135
  prevalence of, 113
  psychotic disorders and, 79,
    100–102
  specialized treatment of,
    125–126

Subsyndromal depressive
  symptoms, prevalence of in
  elderly, 2
Suicide
  alcohol abuse and, 133,
    134–136
  bipolar disorder and, 86
  comorbid alcoholism and
    depression, 133
Supplemental insurance, and
  Medicare, 152

Tacrine
  Alzheimer's disease and, 52
  depression in dementia and, 13
Tardive dyskinesia, and
  antipsychotics, 77, 84, 103
Tau protein
  Alzheimer's disease and, 44, 58
  dementia with Lewy bodies
    and, 39–40
Thought disorder, and
  schizophrenia, 82
Ticlopidine, and vascular
  dementia, 61
Tolerance, and substance
  dependence, 118–119
Training, financing of in geriatric
  psychiatry, 169–170
Traumatic brain injury (TBI), and
  cognitive rehabilitation,
  63–64. *See also* Head injury
Treatment. *See also* Behavioral
  interventions; Cognitive-
  behavioral therapy;
  Electroconvulsive therapy;
  Psychoactive medications;
  Psychosocial treatments
  of alcohol use, 121–131, 133
  of Alzheimer's disease, 38,
    51–60

of anxiety disorders, 20–22
of benzodiazepine abuse,
130–131
of bipolar disorder, 86–87
of delirium, 96
of delusional disorder, 89
of dementia with Lewy
bodies, 41
of depression in dementia,
9–13
of depression with psychotic
features, 88
of frontotemporal dementias, 43
of late-life depression, 3, 133
of psychotic symptoms in
dementia, 91–92
of schizophrenia, 84–85
of vascular dementia, 61–62
Tricyclic antidepressants (TCAs).
See also Antidepressants
alcohol interactions and, **120**
anxiety disorders and, 20
depression in elderly and, 3
medication-induced psychotic
symptoms and, **101**

Ubiquitin, and Lewy bodies, 39
Unipolar depression, with
psychotic symptoms, 87–88

Vaccine, for Alzheimer's disease,
57–58
Valproic acid, and Alzheimer's
disease, 58
Vascular dementia
pathophysiology of, 60
prevalence of depression in, 5

psychoses associated with, 94
treatment of, 61–62
Vasodilators, and vascular
dementia, 61
Venlafaxine, and anxiety
disorders, 21
Viral encephalitis, and psychotic
symptoms, 97
Visual acuity, and psychoses
associated with Alzheimer's
disease, 93. *See also*
Ophthalmological disorders
Vitamin B
Alzheimer's disease and, 48
vascular dementia and, 62
Vitamin E, and Alzheimer's
disease, 38, 56

Waiver programs, and Medicaid,
167
Weight gain, and atypical
antipsychotics, 102
Withdrawal
alcohol abuse and, 116,
124–125
benzodiazepine abuse and,
130
World War I, and posttraumatic
stress disorder in veterans, 17
World War II, and posttraumatic
stress disorder in veterans,
17, 18–19

Ziprasidone
dosing in elderly, **103**
schizophrenia and, 85
side effects in elderly, 102